The Ambr
Tantra

The Ambrosia Heart Tantra

THE SECRET ORAL TEACHING ON THE EIGHT
BRANCHES OF THE SCIENCE OF HEALING

In Sanskrit: *Amṛta-aṣṭāṅgahṛdayopadeśatantra*
In Tibetan: *bDud rtsi snying po yan lag brgyad pa*
gsang ba man ngag gi rgyud

With annotations
by
Dr. Yeshi Dönden

Translated
by
Jhampa Kelsang

LIBRARY OF TIBETAN WORKS AND ARCHIVES

First Edition 1977
Second Edition 1995

ISBN: 81-85102-92-9

Published by the Library of Tibetan Works and Archives, Dharamsala, H. P. (India) and printed at Indraprastha Press (CBT), 4 Bahadurshah Zafar Marg,, New Delhi 110002.

Contents

PART ONE

The Root Tantra

PART TWO

The Explanatory Tantra

Contents

PART ONE

The Root Tantra

PART TWO

The Explanatory Tantra

Publisher's Note

The Tibetan medical system with its emphasis on natural healing methods has, for centuries, held the position of being an exclusive discipline in Tibetan culture and civilisation. A unique tradition, the Tibetan art of healing has evolved through the evaluation and co-ordination of diverse ancient medical systems, incorporating the finest qualities and ideas from each of them. The result has been a distinct balance and synthesis of concept and practice directed towards the making of a system at once scientific and valid.

In an age where a growing proportion of people are turning to healing through natural processes, this present volume on Tibetan medicine appears at an appropriate time to respond to the growing interest in Tibetan healing traditions. This book contains the translation of *Root tantra* or *rTza-rGyud* (first part of *rGyud-bZhi*) and first half of *Explanatory Tantra* or *bShad-rGyud* (second part of *rGyud-bZhi*) for a medical student according to tradition.

Lucidly written, the work will serve as a useful guide for both novice and adept and for numerous others attracted to the Tibetan way of life. Comments from scholars and medical professionals would be welcome.

The commentator, Dr. Yeshi Dönden is ex-personal physician to His Holiness the Dalai Lama and studied for many years at Men-tse-khang, Lhasa, attended by the best tutelage. He is therefore ideally suited to the intellectual task that he has undertaken. The Library of Tibetan Works and Archives is indebted to Dr. Dönden and to translator Jhampa Kelsang, both of whom have invested long hours of effort in making part of the Tibetan medical system accessible to the world.

Gyatsho Tshering
Director

Mar. 1996

About the Commentator

Dr. Yeshi Dönden was born in Lhasa, the capital city of Tibet, in 1927. His schooling began at the age of six, and two years later he took the novice vows of a Buddhist monk. He began his preliminary studies of medicine when he was nine, and at the age of 13 he was formally admitted to the Astro-Medical Institute (*sMan rtsis khang*) in Lhasa. There he studied for five years under the master physician Khyenrab Norbhu. His internship lasted from the age of 18 until 22. During this time he spent a couple of hours each day at an English hospital in Lhasa, learning the use of hypodermic syringes and the dressing of wounds. For the next 10 years he travelled widely throughout Tibet healing the ill. Then in 1959, the year of the Tibetan uprising, he fled from Tibet to India and settled in Dharamsala two years later. In 1961 he became the personal physician to His Holiness the Dalai Lama and, in the following year, he refounded the Astro-Medical Institute, in Dharamsala. He remained there until 1969, when he began his private practice. He has attended medical conferences in Europe and looks forward to visiting the West again in order to help bring the Tibetan medical tradition before the eyes of Western physicians and the general public.

Translator's Note

In October of 1973, I suggested to Dr. Yeshi Dönden the possibility of our translating Tibetan medical works into English. I had been in close contact with him for the past two years, often in the role of interpreter when Westerners came to speak with him, and had often witnessed the effective results of his medical practice. He enthusiastically agreed that there was a need for such translations, so we set to work immediately. For several hours each week he gave me a word-by-word explanation first of the *Root Tantra* and then the first half of the *Explanatory Tantra*. While giving these lessons, he drew from several commentaries, especially those by the Regent Sangs rgyas rgya mtsho, as well as from his own experience. His annotations have been indented in the translation and also frequently occur in parentheses within the main text. Such additions were often necessary where the manuscript, which is written in verse, is especially obscure.

Following the translation I have included an appendix giving examples of foods bearing the various inherent and secondary qualities referred to in the text. I have also added a glossary of terms that have been newly translated or are not positively identified in the currently available Tibetan-English dictionaries.

Finally, I would like to express my gratitude to Dr. Jeffrey Hopkins and his staff at the University of Virginia for their invaluable assistance in the final preparation of the translation.

Jhampa Kelsang
Dharamsala, India
December 31, 1974

PART ONE

The Root Tantra

Commentary on the Title

'Tantra', in the Buddhist sense of the word is the name of a classification of teachings by Buddha Shakyamuni, and the Tibetan translation of the word means 'lineage'. The teachings contained in this tantra are called 'secret' because they are to be taught only to those who are free of the three kinds of improper attention and possessed of the six proper attitudes. The former three are:

1. having a mind like an upside-down pot, i.e. not paying attention to the teachings.
2. having a mind like a defiled pot, i.e. examining the teachings with many preconceived ideas or with a poor motivation.
3. having a mind like a leaky pot, i.e. forgetting the teachings as soon as one has received them.

The six proper attitudes are:

1. thinking of oneself as being like an ill person.
2. thinking of the teachings as being the medicine.
3. thinking of one's teacher as being the doctor.
4. regarding all the Awakened Ones as supreme beings and thus sound sources of knowledge.
5. wishing for the flourishing of the teachings.
6. having the intention to overcome one's personal faults by practising the teachings.

This tantra has traditionally been an oral teaching and has been passed on through an unbroken lineage of physicians since the time of Buddha Shakyamuni. The eight branches include:

1. general healing of the body
2. treatment of women's ailments
3. treatment of children's ailments
4. treatment of disorders caused by spirits
5. treatment of wounds
6. treatment for poisoning
7. treatment to combat the effects of old age
8. treatment to bring about fertility

Finally, because of the great preciousness of the teachings contained in this tantra, they are likened to the essence of ambrosia, which conquers death and eliminates illness.

CHAPTER ONE

Introduction

Homage to the King of Aquamarine Light and supreme benefactor, the Awakened One, who has attained perfect fulfilment and overcome all obstructions, he who has reached the ultimate reality and become the fully-endowed conqueror who surpasses all bounds.

It was in his manifestation as the Sovereign Healer that Buddha Shakyamuni delivered the following teachings. The body of the Sovereign Healer is the colour of aquamarine, and he is here called the King of Aquamarine Light because the lustre radiating from his body is bright like the sun and disperses the darkness of the three mental poisons—attachment, hatred and bewilderment—and the three types of physical disorders involving wind, bile and phlegm. The name "Awakened One" refers to those who have awakened from the sleep of ignorance and whose wisdom pervades all that may be known. They have attained the perfect fulfilment of understanding as well as all other virtues such as compassion, concentration and equanimity. By overcoming the obstacles to liberation and to supreme enlightenment, they gain direct, full awareness of the ultimate truth that all things exist in a state of inter-dependence and that nothing has its own independent self-nature. Awakened Ones are endowed with the six qualities of:

1. wealth of power
2. pleasing appearance
3. splendour
4. renown
5. surpassing wisdom
6. great vigour

They are conquerors of the four Maras, beings who obstruct the spiritual growth of living beings. These four include:

1. the Mara of mental distortions, who is especially active in the morning and arouses the three poisons—attachment, hatred and bewilderment—in the minds of living beings.
2. the Mara called Son of the Gods, who is active in the afternoon and incites hatred in living creatures.
3. the Mara called Lord of Death, who is active in the evening and arouses jealousy.
4. the Mara of the aggregates which form each living being (e.g. form, feelings, consciousness, etc.), who is active at night and arouses all mental distortions.

The full qualities of the Awakened Ones are inexpressible for they are limitless.

Due to his compassion, those who merely hear the name of this surpassing conqueror who acts for the benefit of living creatures, are protected from the evil states of existence.

This protection is gained only if there is the combination of one's faith in the Awakened Ones with their compassion. The Awakened Ones' compassion for all creatures is always present, and they are further able to benefit living beings by knowing the inclinations and capacities of each one.

Homage to the Aquamarine Light, the Awakened One, the supreme benefactor who dispels the three mental poisons and the three ailments.

Those who, due to their admiration and faith in the Awakened Ones, receive their protection are freed of the three mental poisons and the three types of disorders.

Thus I have spoken at one time:

Whereas most of the recorded discourses of Buddha begin with the words, "Thus I have heard at one time," here it says 'spoken' due to the fact that the one giving the discourse and the one who requested it were both manifestations of Buddha.

In the village of healing, an abode of sages called `Lovely to Behold,' there lies a palace made of the five kinds of precious materials.

This village, a miraculous creation of Buddha Shakyamuni, was located near Bodh Gaya. When it existed, it was the dwelling place of sages, or those who are themselves upright and who remove the faults of others. The five kinds of precious materials are gold, silver, white and red pearls, and lapis-lazuli.

The palace is adorned with a variety of precious jewels of healing which dispel the 404 ailments that arise from disorders of wind, bile, phlegm and combinations of two or more of these humours. [Furthermore, they] cool ailments of heat, warm ailments of cold, pacify the 1,080 obstacles [to good health], and fulfil all needs and desires.

The precious jewels of healing refer to the following :

1. the pure, precious jewels of men, which radiate light of five colours—white, yellow, red, blue and green—and are endowed with the following seven qualities:

   a. they eliminate the harm of poisons
   b. they eliminate the harm of spirits
   c. they eliminate the harm of darkness
   d. they eliminate the harm of swelling
   e. they cool ailments of heat
   f. they warm ailments of cold
   g. they fulfil wishes

2. the pure, precious jewels of gods, which are endowed with the above seven qualities as well as the following four:

   a. gods living in a realm where these jewels exist know where they dwelt in their former life and where they will be born in the next
   b. lightweight
   c. perfectly pure
   d. having the ability to speak

3. the precious jewels of bodhisattvas, which possess all the above 11 qualities as well as the following three:

   a. bodhisattvas bearing such jewels know when other living beings will die and where they will be reborn

b. they also know when the chain of rebirth of others will end
c. furthermore, when teaching Dharma, the message of the Awakened Ones, they are able to express themselves in many ways depending upon the individual capacities of their disciples

To the south of that village rises Thunderbolt Mountain, upon which lies the power of the sun. On it are found pomegranates, Mesua roxburgii (fruit), Piper longum (fruit) and Capsicum annuum, etc—medicines that relieve ailments of cold—and a forest containing medicines that are hot-tasting, sour, salty and endowed with the inherent qualities of heat and acridity. The medicinal roots, trunks, branches, leaves, flowers and fruits have a delicious aroma and pleasing appearance, and wherever the scent of these delightful medicines pervades no ailments of cold may arise.

> The taste of the pomegranate (Punica granatum) is sour, slightly salty and hot. Its inherent qualities are heat, acridity, roughness and oiliness, and its secondary qualities are motility and dryness. The taste of Mesua roxburgii is hot, slightly salty and sour. Its inherent qualities are heat and acridity, and its secondary qualities are fatlessness, dryness and motility. The taste of Piper longum is hot, slightly salty and sour. Its inherent qualities are acridity, roughness, and the quality of a softening agent. Its secondary qualities are warmth and dryness. Capsicum annuum has the hottest of tastes. Its inherent qualities are roughness and lightness, and its secondary qualities are warmth and dryness.

To the north of that village rises Snowclad Mountain, upon which lies the power of the moon. On it are found sandalwood, camphor, aloewood and nim pa, etc.—medicines that relieve ailments of heat—and a forest containing medicines that taste bitter, sweet and astringent and bear the inherent qualities of coolness and softening agents. The medicinal roots, trunks, branches, leaves, flowers and fruits have a delicious aroma and pleasing appearance, and wherever the scent of these delightful medicines pervades no ailment of heat may arise.

> The taste of sandalwood (Santalum album) is astringent

and slightly hot. Its inherent quality is oiliness, and its secondary qualities are warmth, gentleness, dryness and toughness. The taste of camphor is astringent, sweet and bitter. Its inherent qualities are roughness, coolness and lightness, and its secondary quality is toughness. The taste of aloewood is astringent and slightly hot. Its inherent quality is oiliness, and its secondary qualities are warmth, gentleness and dryness. Nim pa has the most bitter of tastes. Its inherent qualities are coolness and that of a softening agent, and its secondary qualities are thinness [of fluids] and pliability.

To the east of that village rises Fragrant Mountain, upon which grows a forest of myrobalan. Its roots cure ailments of the bones, its trunk cures ailments of the flesh, its branches cure ailments of the vessels and ligaments, its bark cures ailments of the skin, its leaves cure ailments of the hollow organs, its flowers cure ailments of the sense organs and its fruit cures ailments of the heart and other solid organs. At the tops of the five kinds of myrobalan [trees] ripen [fruits] endowed with six tastes, eight inherent qualities, three properties as they pass through the digestive tract and all the 17 secondary qualities. They cure all kinds of illness, and wherever the scent of this fragrant, lovely and pleasing medicine pervades, none of the 404 ailments may arise.

Upon this mountain the power of the sun and moon were equal. The six hollow organs include:

1. the stomach
2. the large intestine
3. the gall bladder
4. the small intestine
5. the urinary bladder
6. the vesicle of regenerative nutriment

The five solid organs include:

1. the lungs
2. the heart
3. the liver
4. the spleen
5. the kidneys

The five kinds of myrobalan trees are:

1. the five-cornered fearless myrobalan
2. yellow myrobalan
3. dry myrobalan
4. shathub ambrosia myrobalan
5. the round-loader myrobalan

The above curing properties of the roots, trunk, etc. refer to all five kinds of myrobalan. Some kinds of myrobalan fruit have all of the six tastes, whereas others have only two or three. The six tastes are:

1. sweet
2. bitter
3. sour
4. salty
5. astringent
6. hot

The eight inherent qualities are:

1. heaviness
2. oiliness
3. coolness
4. softening agent
5. lightness
6. roughness
7. heat
8. acridity

These eight are possessed by all five kinds of myrobalan, for the skin, flesh, upper and lower parts of each fruit have different qualities. The three properties which appear after the fruit has entered the digestive tract are:

1. a sour taste while in the upper region of the stomach, at which time it cures phlegm ailments
2. a salty taste while in the lower region of the stomach, at which time it cures wind ailments
3. a sweet taste while in the blood system, at which time it cures bile ailments

The 17 secondary qualities are:

1. gentleness
2. heaviness
3. warmth
4. oiliness
5. firmness
6. coolness
7. softening agent
8. coldness
9. pliability
10. thinness [of fluids]
11. dryness
12. fatlessness
13. heat
14. lightness
15. acridity
16. roughness
17. motility

The inherent qualities of a substance are those that remain unaffected by most chemical processes, whereas its secondary qualities may readily be changed. For example, heaviness is an inherent quality of raw sugar, and it remains even when the sugar is refined. On the other hand, warmth, one of the secondary qualities of raw sugar, changes to coolness due to the refining process.

To the west of that village rises Cool Mountain, upon which grow the six good medicines. There are also found the five kinds of cong. zhi, which cure all ailments, the five kinds of brag.zhun, the five kinds of medicinal water, and the five types of hot springs.

Upon this mountain the power of the sun and moon were equal. The six good medicines are:

1. bamboo manna (a substance secreted from the joints of bamboo)
2. saffron
3. clove
4. nutmeg
5. cardamom (Elettaria cardamomum)
6. ka.ko.la

The five kinds of cong.zhi (a kind of stone) are:

1. male
2. female
3. son
4. daughter
5. neuter

The five kinds of brag.zhun are:

1. gold zhun
2. silver zhun
3. copper zhun
4. iron zhun
5. lead zhun

Brag.zhun is the 'sweat' that arises from these minerals when the weather is very hot and dry. The five kinds of medicinal water are those that cure:

1. phlegm disorders
2. bile disorders
3. wind disorders
4. disorders of any two of the three humours
5. disorders of all three humours

The five kinds of hot springs are those containing:

1. rdo.sol and cong.zhi
2. rdo.sol, cong.zhi and sulphur
3. rdo.sol and sulphur
4. rdo.sol and brag.zhun
5. rdo.sol, brag.zhun, ldong.ros and sulphur

All around the village are mountain meadows of saffron from which arise the fragrance of incense. There are medicinal minerals and salts to be found in all the stones. On the treetops in this forest of healing, peacocks, cranes, parrots and other fowl burst forth with melodious song, and on the ground dwell all kinds of creatures bearing good medicines, such as elephants, bears and musk deer. [The region] is adorned by all types of healing agents that grow or may be found [on earth].

On an aquamarine throne in the centre of the palace sat the Master, the Blessed One, the supreme benefactor and healer known as the King of Aquamarine Light. The Master was completely surrounded by four circles of disciples—gods, sages, non-Buddhists and Buddhists. The circle of gods included the divine physician Kyegü Dagpo Nyurwa, the divine physician Thakar, the divine sovereign Indra and the goddess Dütsima. These and many other divine disciples were congregated there. The circle of sages included the great sage Son of Gyünshé, Mezhin Jug, Mukhyü Dsin, Son of Dokyong, Sholdo Kyé, Kanyi Chö, Thangla Bar and Nabso Kyé. These and many other sages were gathered there. The circle of non-Buddhists included the patriarch of non-Buddhists, Brahma, Mahadeva, Shri Ralpachen, Vishnu and Zhönnu Dongdhug. These and many other non-Buddhists were gathered there. The circle of Buddhists included the glorious Manjushri, the powerful Avalokiteshvara, Vajrapani, Ananda and the physician Zhönnu. These and many other Buddhists were gathered there.

In his manifestation as the Sovereign Healer, Buddha appears in his richly adorned Sambhogakaya form, which is the way the Awakened Ones appear to those of high spiritual development. The palm of his right hand faces out, symbolizing his bestowal of protection, and in it he holds the fruit of the myrobalan tree, showing that he gives protection from illness. In his left hand he holds a bowl containing the three kinds of ambrosia:

1. ambrosia that cures disease and has the power to bring one back from death
2. ambrosia that counteracts aging
3. never-depleting ambrosia that increases concentration and understanding

The circle of gods included those followers of Buddha dwelling in any of the three realms of desire, form and formlessness. Among the circle of sages were those with matted hair and emaciated, naked bodies and ascetics who lived on fruit, slept under a blanket of leaves at night and wore clothing of bark during the day. Among the circle of non-Buddhists were divine beings carrying white conches and tridents, some having four faces and others wearing their hair twisted on top of their head. The circle of Buddhists included: Manjushri, who is the Vajra* body of all the Awakened Ones and is the embodiment of their wisdom; Avalokiteshvara, who is the Vajra speech of all the Awakened Ones and is the embodiment

---

* The Vajra is a symbol of power and immutability.

of their love and compassion; Vajrapani, who is the Vajra mind of all the Awakened Ones and is the embodiment of their power; Buddha Shakyamuni's disciple Ananda, and many other physicians.

At that time, each of the four types of disciples understood the words of the Master to be of the tradition of its own master. This [the following] is called the "Tradition of the Sage", for such is one who is free of faults of the body, speech and mind, upright and true, and who corrects the faults present in others.

The fact that the individual disciples who received this teaching were able to understand it as being of their own tradition is due to the Buddhas' unique ability to teach all those who seek their guidance effectively. The teachings about to be related here are those heard by Sage Yilé Kyé, who has the nature of the Buddhas' discriminating wisdom. It was he who requested the Sovereign Healer to teach the four tantras on medicine, and he himself was a manifestion of the Buddhas' speech. Thus he is here referred to as 'the Sage', for he is free of all mental defilements and physical imbalances.

CHAPTER TWO
Enumeration of Subjects to be Discussed

At that time the Master Buddha, the King of Aquamarine Light, who is the supreme benefactor and healer, entered the mental absorption called `The Sovereign Healer, Who Pacifies the 404 Ailments'. As soon as he entered meditation, many rays of multicoloured light spread forth from his heart to all the 10 directions, clearing away the mental defilements of all animate beings of the 10 directions and pacifying all ailments of the three mental poisons, which arise from ignorance. Then upon drawing them [the light rays] back to his heart, the illusory form of Buddha, named Sage Rigpé Yeshé emanated from his mind.

> The defilements of the mind which were dispelled by the light rays refer to the three unwholesome characteristics of the mind, namely, covetousness, malice and grasping at mistaken beliefs. The 10 directions include the eight points of the compass and the directions up and down. As soon as the light rays returned to his heart, there came forth from the omniscient mind one having the nature of the Buddhas' mirror-like wisdom, or the Immovable Vajra, known by the name of Sage Rigpé Yeshé.

Appearing in the sky before him, he spoke these words of introduction to the sagacious disciples: "O friends! This you should know! One who desires to remain free of illness and to cure illness should learn the oral teaching on the science of healing. One who desires long life should learn the oral teaching on the science of healing. One who desires to receive religious teaching, wealth and happiness should learn the oral teaching on the science of healing. One who desires to free anyone from the suffering of illness and who desires the respect of others should learn the oral teaching on the science of healing." Having spoken thus, many rays of multicoloured light spread forth from the tongue of Buddha, the King of Aquamarine Light, to all the 10 directions, clearing away the verbal defilements of all animate beings of the 10 directions and pacifying all illness and spirits. Then upon drawing them back to his tongue, the emanation of the Buddhas' speech named Sage Yilé Kyé appeared, prostrating himself before the Awakened One and circumambulating him. Then in the manner of a lion he spoke these words of request before the Awakened One on behalf of the sagacious disciples: "O Master, Sage Rigpé Yeshé! As we desire to obtain this bounty for the sake of ourselves and others, how may we learn the oral teaching on the science of healing?"

> Sage Rigpé Yeshé addressed the circle of disciples first, because they were left speechless by the glory of Buddha's countenance and so were unable to request teachings. The verbal defilements spoken of here refer to the four unwholesome kinds of speech—lying, slander, harsh speech and senseless speech. As soon as the light rays returned to Buddha's tongue, there came forth from the omniscient mind one having the nature of the Buddhas' discriminating wisdom, or Boundless Light, known by the name of Sage Yilé Kyé. He prostrated thrice before the Sovereign Healer, then circumambulated him three times. Having done so, he fearlessly knelt before the Awakened One, placing his right knee upon the ground and with palms pressed together, requested that teaching be given in order to fulfil the desires of all the disciples.

Having spoken thus, the emanation of [Buddha's] mind, Sage Rigpé Yeshé, gave this reply: "O great sages! Learn the Oral Tradition Tantra on the science of healing. Learn the branches. Learn the divisions. Learn the compilations. Learn the chapters." Then Sage Yilé Kyé asked: "O Master, how may we learn the Oral Tradition Tantra on the science of healing?" The Master replied: "Learn the four tantras—the Root Tantra, the Explanatory Tantra, the Oral Tradition Tantra and the Subsequent Tantra. These are known as the four tantras.

"What are the eight branches to be learned? They are: (1) physical ailments, (2) children's ailments, (3) women's ailments, (4) men's ailments, (5) [ailments caused by] spirits, (6) [wounds inflicted by] weapons, (7) [disorders of the] aged and (8) sterility. These are known as the eight branches.

"The 11 principles to be learned are as follows: (1) the principle of the synthesis of the fundamentals, (2) the principle of the existence of the body [dealing with the transformation of the body from conception to death], (3) the principle of the rise and decline of illness, (4) the principle of behaviour, (5) the principle of nutrition, (6) the principle of preparing medicine [and their individual tastes and secondary qualities], (7) the principle of using [medical] instruments, (8) the principle of remaining free of common illness [and signs of age], (9) the principle of the characteristics of diagnosis, (10) the principle of the methods of healing and (11) the principle of the [required physical, verbal and mental] behaviour of a physician. These are known as the 11 principles.

"The 15 divisions to be learned are the following : (1) the division on curing the three disorders [of wind, bile and phlegm and their combinations], (2) the division on curing stomach disorders, (3) the division on curing heat disorders, (4) the division on healing the upper portion of the body [from the navel up], (5) the division on healing (five) solid organs and (six) hollow organs, (6) the division on healing the genitals [both male and female], (7) the division on curing miscellaneous disorders, (8) the division on healing wounds arising from disorders within the body, (9) the division on healing children, (10) the division on curing women's ailments, (11) the division on curing disorders caused by spirits, (12) the division on healing wounds inflicted by weapons, (13) the division on curing disorders caused by poisoning, (14) the division on healing the aged [and combatting the aging process] and (15) the division on inducing fertility. These are known as the 15 divisions.

"The four compilations to be studied are as follows: (1) the compilation on the examination of the pulse and urine, (2) the compilation on the [preparation and individual properties of] medicines used in internally curing disorders, (3) the compilation of methods of evacuation [of the source of the disorder from the body, e.g. by inducing vomiting or evacuation of the bowels] and (4) the compilation of gentle [e.g. applying hot towels to the skin] and rough [e.g. burning and surgery] types of treatment. These are known as the four compilations."

> The eight branches are covered in all the four tantras, particularly in the Root Tantra. The 11 principles are dealt with in the Explanatory Tantra, the 15 divisions in the Oral Tradition Tantra, the four compilations in the Subsequent Tantra, and the 156 chapters are found in all the four tantras.

The 156 chapters to be studied are listed as follows: the six chapters including: (1) the introduction, (2) [the enumeration of] subjects to be discussed, (3) the basis [of illness], (4) diagnosis [of disorders], (5) methods of healing and (6) the enumeration [of metaphors with regard to parts of the body, illnesses, etc.]. These are known as the Root Tantra, in which the fundamentals [of medicine] are compiled.

The 11 principles are contained in the following chapters of the Explanatory Tantra: (1) the synthesis of the Explanatory [Tantra], (2) the manner of the formation [of the body during gestation], (3) similes [for the body], (4) anatomy, (5) the characteristics [of the body], (6) the classifications [of different types of bodies, e.g. those especially prone to wind disorders], (7) the signs of death, (8) the causes of illnesses, (9) the conditions contributing to illnesses, (10) the manner of entrance [of illnesses], (11) the characteristics [of illnesses], (12) the classification [of illnesses], (13) [medical advice on healthy] daily behaviour, (14) [medical advice on healthy] seasonal behaviour, (15) [medical advice on healthy] behaviour on the occasions [of specific activities], (16) the way to eat [discussing the benefits and harm of different kinds of food], (17) foods [and food combinations] to be avoided, (18) the appropriate amount of food to be eaten, (19) the tastes [and digestive qualities] of medicines, (20) the inherent qualities [of different kinds of medicines], (21) [a concise explanation on] how to prepare medicines, (22) medical instruments, (23) [how to] remain free of illness, (24) direct diagnosis of [the three types of] disorders, (25) the deceptive, faulty means of diagnosis [of asking the patient about his illness and his recent activities prior to the illness], (26) diagnosis with regard to the four classifications [of illness] which may or may not be cured, (27) general healing methods, (28) specific healing methods, (29) two methods of healing, (30) [a still clearer explanation of] actual methods of healing, and (31) [the required behaviour of a] physician. There are three single [or unrelated chapters—ch. 22, 23 and 31], four [groups of] three [related chapters—ch. 13-15, 16-18, 19-21 and 24-26], [one group of] four [related chapters—ch. 27-30], [one group of] five [related chapters—ch. 8-12], [one group of] six (related chapters—ch. 2-7) and the first chapter of compilation—all totalling 31 chapters.

The 15 divisions are contained in the following chapters of the Oral Tradition Tantra: (1) [the manner in which this teaching was] requested; [the different types of disorders; their treatment and the action to be followed by the patient with regard to:] (2) wind disorders, (3) bile disorders, (4) phlegm disorders and (5) combinations [of the above three]; the six chapters on [treating stomach disorders and other] chronic ailments [arising therefrom], (6) disorders of digestion, (7) formation of stones [in the stomach, intestines, etc.], (8) a disorder involving swelling of the head in the morning and legs in the evening, (9) a disorder involving swelling of the side of the body facing down when sleeping, (10) abdominal swelling and (11) the kind of tuberculosis that results in coughing and thinness [this variety is difficult to cure, because if, for example, medication for the cough is given, it causes disorder in the stomach]; the 16 chapters [on treating heat disorders], (12) a general [explanation of] heat disorders, (13) illness such that the pulse and urine indicate a cold disorder, while there is actually a heat disorder, or vice versa, (14) [treatment to be given] after a heat disorder has been rectified, (15) rising heat disorders [which can only be cured by first letting them rise to their peak], (16) very high heat disorders, (17) heat disorders which [for some reason, e.g. a sudden change in environment or climate], are not able to rise to their peak; [this type is called 'hollow', for it is similar to a hollow wheat kernel on a stalk that has grown too fast], (18) hidden heat disorders [such that the body seems externally to be suffering from a cold disorder], (19) chronic heat disorders, (20) heat disorders due to the mixing of blood and lymph, (21) heat disorders that pervade the entire body, (22) heat disorders having the nature of the disorders of bile, (23) contagious heat disorders [these began to increase in prevalence during the 17th and 18th centuries and are most common in this century; they are caused by engine exhaust in the air], (24) [the six kinds of] poxes, (25) dysentery, (26) the very dangerous illness involving] swelling of the arms and legs or the throat and (27) [the many varieties of] the common cold; the six chapters on [treating the various disorders in] the upper portion of the body: (28) the head, (29) the eyes, (30) the ears, (31) the nose, (32) the mouth [including the teeth, lips, etc.] and (33) the throat; the eight chapters on [treating disorders of] the solid organs and hollow organs: (34) the heart, (35) the lungs, (36) the liver, (37) the spleen, (38) the kidneys, (39) the stomach, (40) the small intestine and (41) the large intestine; [treating] disorders of the genitals: (42) male and (43) female; the 19 chapters on [treating] miscellaneous disorders: (44) blockage of the throat passage, (45) stoppage of food in the canal before it reaches the stomach, (46) thirst, (47) hiccoughs, (48) asthma, (49) stomach pain arising from being suddenly chilled while still wet with perspiration, (50) disorders involving organisms [in the stomach, intestines, etc.], (51) vomiting, (52) diarrhoea, (53) blockage of air in the stomach combined with an inability to defecate, (54) blockage of the urinary canal [e.g. by stones], (55) obstinate urinary disorders, (56) disorders involving both diarrhoea and heat, (57) gout, (58) disorders involving dryness of the limbs and ligaments such that the hands become twisted, (59) disorders of the lymphatic system involving itching and dryness of the skin, (60) disorders involving trembling and an inability to bend the neck or limbs, (61) skin disorders and (62) subtle disorders; the eight chapters on [treating] wounds arising from disorders within the body: (63) wounds which are small at first, then enlarge, becoming difficult to heal, (64) haemorrhoids, (65) a disorder arising from impurity of the blood of resulting in large red itching sores from which blood emerges if scratched, (66) cancerous sores [not of the most dangerous variety] occurring in such organs as the heart, stomach and liver, (67) the many varieties of cancer-like tumours, (68) swelling of the testicles, (69) disorders arising from the descent of blood and lymph from the upper to the lower portion of the body, resulting in extremely painful swelling of the legs, and (70) a rare disorder involving first swelling, then the emergence of pus and finally the appearance of a hole between the anus and genitals; the three chapters on [healing] children: (71) various types of treatment related to children [e.g. medicine to be taken by women after sexual intercourse and prior to the next menstruation to cause the coming child to be male, and medicine to be taken by pregnant women to safeguard the life of the child in the womb], (72) children's ailments and (73) disorders caused by spirits while the child is sleeping; the three chapters on [treating] women's disorders: (74) women's disorders in general, (75) specific disorders and (76) common disorders of women; the five chapters on [treating] disorders caused by spirits: (77) a variety of disorders caused by one classification of spirit, (78) mental disorder such that one is unaware of one's actions, due to the mind's being under the control of a spirit, (79) mental disorder such that one remains with eyes fixed, unthinking and unresponsive, (80) disorders caused by planetary influences [e.g. paralysis of one side of the body, dumbness or fits such that one's mouth becomes contorted, the eyes staring upwards and the fists clenched] and (81) disorders caused by Nagas, a kind of creature invisible to humans but which often takes the form of a snake [they cause harm by breathing on people, which usually results in swelling or disorders of the lymphatic system]; the five chapters on [treating externally inflicted] wounds: (82) general treatment of wounds, (83) head wounds [of all kinds], (84) throat wounds, (85) wounds on the upper and lower trunk and (86) the limbs; the three chapters on [treating] disorders caused by poisoning: (87) disorders due to manufactured poisons [e.g. poisoning through eating food that has been sprayed with insecticides], (88) poisoning from unhealthy combinations of food and (89) disorders due to natural poisons [e.g. from certain flowers, snakes, spiders, rabid animals, etc.]; (90) treatment for the aged [for longevity and rejuvenation], using medicine containing essential nutriment; [methods to induce] fertility by (91) treating the sperm and (92) [causing] the woman to be able to give birth.

Thus there is one single chapter (ch. 90), two pairs (ch. 42-3 and 91-2), three groups of three (ch. 74-6, 87-9 and 71-3), one group of four (ch. 2-5), two groups of five (ch. 77-81 and 82-6), two groups of six (ch. 28-33 and 6-11), two groups of eight (ch. 63-70 and 34-41), one group of 16 (ch. 12-27) and one group of 19 (ch. 44-62). These plus the [chapter of] requesting make a total of 92.

The four compilations are contained in the following chapters of the Subsequent Tantra: (1) [examination of] the pulse, (2) [examination of] the urine; [the classification, individual healing properties and manner of preparation of:] (3) decoctions, (4) powdered medicines, (5) pills, (6) syrups, (7) medicinal oils, (8) calcinated powders [made from gold, silver, copper and other metals], (9) desiccated powders [medicines composed of the solidification of the fluid strained from the boiled mixture of a variety of ingredients], (10) alcoholic medicines [especially used in treating wind disorders], (11) [medicines made from many kinds of] precious materials [e.g. pearl, gold, silver and gems], (12) medicine prepared solely from plants, (13) medicine prepared from oils [either to be taken orally or to be applied to the skin], (14) [medicine to cause] motion in the two excretory channels, (15) [medicine to induce] vomiting, (16) medicine to be poured into the nostrils, (17) pills which are to be inserted into the anus, (18) medicine which is mixed with water, then inserted into the anus in order to cause bowel motion, (19) medicine to cause a flow of urine [used to clean the vessels and to discharge kidney stones], (20) the method of blood-letting, (21) the method of cauterization, (22) the method of applying hot water, cloths or cold stones on the skin, (23) ointment to be applied to the skin in cases of wounds or swelling, (24) ointments used primarily in treating skin diseases and (25) surgical methods.

[Among these chapters] there is one pair (ch. 1-2), one group of 10 (ch. 3-12), one group of seven (ch. 3-9) and one group of six (ch. 20-25).

Thus the Root Tantra has six chapters, the Explanatory Tantra has 31, the Oral Tradition Tantra has 92 chapters and the Subsequent Tantra has 25chapters, bringing the total for the four tantras to 154. [In addition], there is the concluding chapter [of praise of the four tantras] and the chapter explaining the qualities required of a student to whom these tantras may be taught [e.g. compassion and intelligence], making a total of 156. They fall into the eight branches as follows: 70 [chapters] on the [general healing of the] body, six on children's and women's ailments [three each], three on [the treatment of cases of] poisoning, five on [disorders caused by] spirits, five on [the treatment of] wounds, one on [the use of] essential nutriment [used for rejuvenation] and two on [treatment to bring about] fertility. These chapters are found throughout the [latter] three tantras.

CHAPTER THREE

The Basis of Illness

Then Sage Yilé Kyé asked Sage Rigpé Yeshé: "O Master, Sage Rigpé Yeshé, of the four kinds of tantras on the science of healing, how may we learn the Root Tantra? May the physician, the Sovereign Healer, explain." Then the emanation of [Buddha's] mind, Sage Rigpé Yeshé, replied: "O great sage Yilé Kyé! First I shall illustrate the collection of the main points of the Root Tantra. About three roots are coiled nine trunks. [From these] spread forth 47 branches, [and on these grow] 224 leaves and ripen five clear flowers and fruits. These are said to be the total of [the main points of] the Root Tantra.

"I shall elaborate further. There are the three classifications of humours, bodily constituents and impurities. Their balance and imbalance [correspondingly] cause the body to thrive or to be overcome. The humours are wind, bile and phlegm. The five kinds of wind are: (1) life-supporting, (2) upward-moving, (3) pervasive, (4) fire-accompanying and (5) downward-clearing. The five kinds of bile are: (1) digestive, (2) colour-transforming, (3) accomplishing, (4) visually-operating and (5) complexion-clearing. The five types of phlegm are: (1) supportive, (2) mixing, (3) experiencing, (4) satisfying and (5) connecting. The bodily constituents include: (1) chyle, (2) blood, (3) flesh, (4) fat, (5) bone, (6) marrow and (7) regenerative fluid [for both sexes]. The impurities include: (1) excrement, (2) urine and (3) perspiration. Thus if all of these 25 are in balance and the three factors of the tastes and inherent qualities [of one's food] and one's behaviour [are wholesome, one's health and life] will flourish. If they are not, [one's health and life] will be harmed. Illnesses are produced by three causes [aided by] four contributing circumstances, [resulting in their] meeting the six types of entrances, then remaining in the upper, lower and middle portions of the body. Along the 15 pathways [imbalances of the humours] increase in accordance with the nine [conditions falling within the categories of] age, environment and time. There are nine [situations of which the] result is certain death and 12 types of reaction-imbalances [of the three humours]. [All] these factors fall into the two [categories of] heat and cold.

"Thus with regard to the 63 illnesses to be healed, attachment, hatred and bewilderment are the three causes consecutively producing imbalances of wind, bile and phlegm. Along with these, the four contributing circumstances of time [e.g. wearing light clothes in the winter], spirits, food [in improper quantities or combinations] and behaviour, cause [the humours] to increase and decrease [e.g. wearing light clothing when chilled causes the wind to increase and the bile to decrease]. [The imbalance then] spreads over the skin, increases in the flesh, moves along the vessels, meets the bones and descends upon the solid and hollow organs.

"Phlegm depends upon the brain and remains in the upper portion of the body. Bile depends on the lining of the liver and remains in the middle portion of the body. Wind depends upon the hip-bones and the base of the spine and remains in the lower portion of the body.

"The pathways of wind, bile and phlegm [disorders among the categories of] the bodily constituents, impurities, sense organs and solid and hollow organs are said to be the following: [the pathways ways of wind disorders are] the bones, ears, nerves under the skin, the heart, the vital channel and the large intestine. [The pathways of bile disorders are:] chyle, flesh, fat, marrow, regenerative fluid, excrement, urine, the nose, tongue, lungs, spleen, stomach, kidneys and urinary bladder.

"People advanced in age are 'wind people' [for they are especially prone to disorders of the wind], those of middle age are 'bile people', and young people [up to the age of 16 or so] are 'phlegm people'. These are the dangers of age groups.

"Cold and windy places are said to be 'regions of wind' [i.e. disorders of wind are especially common there], oppressively hot, dry places are 'regions of bile', and damp, oily places are 'regions of phlegm'.

"Wind disorders arise [particularly] in the summer, in the evening and just before dawn. Bile disorders arise in the autumn, in the afternoon and at night, and phlegm disorders arise in the spring, at twilight and at dawn.

"The nine maladies of which the result is certain death are said to be the following: (1) the depletion of the three factors supporting life [namely, one's 'life karma', i.e. the mental imprints from acts in the previous lifetimes which determine the duration of one's life; one's merit, or positive mental imprints resulting from wholesome acts in the past; and a relationship from past lives with a physician from whom one may receive effective treatment], (2) disorders which increase regardless of the medicine taken, (3) disorders which cannot be effectively counteracted regardless of the treatment given, (4) the piercing of the solid organs [by weapons and so forth], (5) a wind disorder advanced to such a degree that the patient is no longer able to breathe, (6) a heat disorder having risen beyond the point of possible cure, (7) a cold disorder having fallen beyond the point of possible cure, (8) inability of the bodily constituents to function properly and (9) the point when the harm of a spirit has taken full effect.

"The 12 types of reaction-imbalances are: disturbance in the balance of (1) bile and (2) phlegm after curing a wind disorder; imbalance of (3) bile and (4) phlegm while still treating a wind disorder; imbalance of (5) wind and (6) phlegm after curing a bile disorder and (7 and 8) while still treating it; imbalance of (9) wind and (10) bile after curing a phlegm disorder and (11 and 12) while still treating it.

"[All imbalances of] wind and phlegm are [in the category of] cold [disorders] and [are likened to] water. [All ailments of] the blood and bile are [in the category of] heat [disorders] and are [likened to] fire. [Ailments due to] worms [or any organisms in the body] and lymph (disorders) are common to both heat and cold [disorders].

"By knowing the above eight categories, one understands all the characteristics involved in physical disorders."

CHAPTER FOUR

Diagnosis and Symptoms

Then Sage Rigpé Yeshé spoke these words: "O great sage, listen! All may be known about illness through observation, touch [i.e. feeling the pulse] and questioning [the patient about his illness]. Visual observation refers to examining the tongue and urine. This diagnosis involves understanding a visual object. The contact of the fingers [with the pulse] is the source of communication [from within the body, i.e. it is the means by which the physician learns of the inner conditions of the patient's body]. The diagnosis [of the pulse] involves understanding the object of examination [i.e. understanding what these 'messages' sent from within the body mean]. One verbally asks [the patient] about the conditions which led to the arising of [his] illness, the symptoms of the illness and about his diet [i.e. what food he ate prior to the illness, what he eats at present and how this food affects him]. This diagnosis involves hearing and understanding [the patient's] voice.

"The tongue of a [person with a] wind disorder is red, dry [at night] and rough. The tongue of a [person with a] bile disorder is thickly covered with a light-yellow film of phlegm. [The tongue of a person with] a phlegm disorder is [completely coated with] a light film [of phlegm] and is pale, soft and wet.

"The urine of [a person with] a wind disorder is like water and has much froth. The urine of [a person with] a bile disorder is orange, has much vapour and an unpleasant odour. The urine of [a person with] a phlegm disorder is clear and has little odour or vapour.

"The pulse of [a person with] a wind disorder is resilient [in that it goes down when the vessels are firmly pressed and returns when the pressure is removed] and sometimes stops momentarily. The pulse of [a person with] a bile disorder is fast, strong and tight [like a twisted thread]. The pulse of [a person with] a phlegm disorder is hardly noticeable, weak and slow.

"[With respect to] questioning, the conditions contributing [to a wind disorder] are light and rough foods [e.g. black coffee] and behaviour [such as going without sleep, staying in a windy place or experiencing much suffering]. [Symptoms of wind disorders are] yawning, trembling, stretching, shivering, [pain in] the hip joints, base of the spine and all the joints, randomly moving, randomly appearing shooting pains, dry heaves, dullness of the senses and unsteadiness of the mind. [Symptoms of wind] disorders [are mostly evident] when one is hungry. Oily and highly nutritious foods are of certain benefit [to a person with these symptoms].

"Acrid and hot foods [e.g. alcohol] and behaviour [e.g. violent or disturbing action and remaining under a hot sun] contribute to [bile disorders, which have the symptoms of] a bitter taste in the mouth, headache, hotness of the body and shooting pains in the upper body. [These symptoms are strongest] while food is being digested, and [such a patient] is benefitted by cool [foods and environment]. Heavy and oily foods and behaviour [such as lying for a long time on moist earth] contribute to [phlegm disorders, which have the symptoms of] an uncomfortable [full] feeling in the stomach, difficulty in digesting food, food coming up [again and again] from the stomach, inability to taste food, protrusion of the stomach, [frequent, bad smelling] belches, heaviness of the body and mind, coldness [of the body] both internally and externally and discomfort [directly] after eating. Warm food and environment give relief [to a person with these symptoms].

"By means of the above 38 methods of diagnosis, one is able to correctly determine with certainty [the nature of] all illnesses."

CHAPTER FIVE

Methods of Healing

Then Sage Rigpé Yeshé spoke these words: "O great sage, listen! There are four remedies that heal illness: (1) food, (2) behaviour, (3) medicine and (4) external medical treatment.

(1) "The foods [prescribed] for one with a wind disorder are: horse meat, donkey meat, the flesh of a marmot, aged dried meat, human flesh, grain oil, aged butter, dark brown sugar, garlic, onion, [fresh warm] milk [directly from the cow], beer made from barley mixed with the two medicines Ica and mnye, liquor made from brown sugar and liquor made from ground bone.

"The foods [prescribed] for one with a bile disorder are: curd [made from cow's or goat's milk], the remainder after removing the butter from curd, fresh butter, game meat, goat meat, meat from a thin type of cow [in Tibetan called skom], fresh ground barley, spinach, a vegetable named khur tshod, black tea, spring water, water from melted snow and water that has cooled after boiling.

"One with a phlegm disorder should eat the following: mutton, wild yak meat, flesh from carnivorous mammals, fish, honey, roasted barley flour [made from aged barley grown in a dry region], curd made from yak's milk, the remainder after the butter has been removed from the curd of yak's milk, thick [aged] beer and boiled water which is still hot.

(2) "One with a wind disorder should stay in a warm place and be with pleasant friends. One with a bile disorder should stay in a cool place and not exert himself. One with a phlegm disorder should be very active [e.g. do physical exercises or take walks] and stay in a warm place.

(3) "Medicines for a person with a wind disorder are: sweet [e.g. medicine made from brown sugar], sour [e.g. made from aged beer], salty [e.g. made from sea salt], [and have the inherent qualities of] oiliness [e.g. made from black aloewood], heaviness [e.g. made from black salt] and gentleness [e.g. made from the kandakari tree].

"Medicines for a person with a bile disorder are: sweet [e.g. made from grapes], bitter [e.g. made from Hemerocallis minor], thick [of fluids, e.g. made from white sandalwood], [and having the inherent qualities of] coolness [e.g. made from camphor], thinness [e.g. made from the tree Pterospermum acerifolium] and a softening agent [e.g. made from bamboo manna, a substance secreted in the joints of bamboo].

"Medicines for a person with a phlegm disorder are: hot [e.g. made from the fruit of the tree Mesua roxburgii], sour [e.g. made from Crataegus sanguinea], [and have the inherent qualities of] acridity [e.g. made from sal-ammoniac], roughness [e.g. made from the berries of the shrub Hippophae rhamnoides] and lightness [e.g. made from Capsicum annuum].

"There are two [methods of treatment] which are combined with these tastes and inherent qualities, [namely,] pacification and cleansing. [With the former, the patient takes medicine and the disturbance or disorder in his body is pacified. With the latter, medicine is taken to induce vomiting or evacuation of the bowels, thereby ridding the body of the cause of the disorder.]

"The pacifying treatment for wind disorders involves liquid [medicine that is to be drunk] and medicinal oils. For bile disorders it involves decoctions and powdered medicines, and for phlegm disorders pills and powdered medicines called tres sam [are used].

"The liquid medicines include: liquid made from bones [specifically, bone joints of mammals, which are ground up and made into a liquid], the four nutriments [one of which is prepared by boiling brown sugar into water, then pouring it into aged beer and adding salt] and water in which an old dried sheep's head has been boiled.

"The medicinal oils include [individual medicines made primarily from the following ingredients:] nutmeg, garlic, the three fruits (Terminalia chebula, Crataegus sanguinea and Crataegus pinnatifida), the 'five roots' and [a kind of poison called] sman chen.

"The decoctions include [individual medicines made primarily from the following ingredients:] ma nu, sle tres, Gentiana barbata and the [three] fruits.

"The powdered medicines include [individual medicines made primarily from the following ingredients:] camphor, [white] sandalwood, saffron and bamboo manna.

"The types of pills include [individual medicines made primarily from the following ingredients;] btsan dug and various kinds of salts.

"The types of tres sam include [individual medicines made primarily from the following ingredients:] pomegranate, Rhododendron anthopogonoides maxim, rgod ma kha (a very hot medicine), [various kinds of] salts and cong zhi. These powdered medicines warm [the body].

"The cleansing treatment for wind disorders involves the use of enemas, for bile, purgatives and for phlegm, inducing vomiting. The types of enemas include the following: an enema that is first inserted into the anus, then the patient claps his feet together to make the medicine go up the tract; an enema that is first inserted into the anus, after which the patient is held upside-down and shaken to make the medicine go up the tract; and an enema called bkru ma slen. Purgation involves: medicine to be taken as preparation; medicine with a very unpleasant odour and taste which is taken orally and directly causes purgation; the rough method [of drinking much hot water after taking the above medicine to prevent vomiting, meanwhile holding a cold bottle of water or cold towels against the throat for the same purpose]; and the gentle method [of holding a hot-water bottle or hot towels against the abdomen to prevent pain and to cause a slower evacuation of the bowels]. Inducing vomiting involves: the rough method [of sitting on one's heels with the thighs pressed against the abdomen after taking the medicine. In this position one vomits]; and the gentle method [of keeping very warm after vomiting in order to prevent other disorders from arising as an after-effect of the treatment].

"Methods [used in treating wind disorders include:] [the application of the ointment] bsku mnye [which is made primarily from sesamum oil] and the Mongolian method of cauterization [which involves mixing cumin seed oil with salt and wrapping this mixture in a cloth. The cloth is then dipped into hot butter and applied to the surface of the skin].

"[Methods used in treating bile disorders include:] the inducement of perspiration [by wrapping blankets around the patient], blood-letting [e.g. when the blood pressure is very high], and having the patient stand naked under a cold waterfall.

"[Methods used in treating phlegm disorders include:] wrapping cloths dipped in boiling water on the body, especially around the abdomen, and cauterization [with gold, silver or copper-tipped instruments].

"If one uses the above 98 methods of healing with care and respect, freedom from the swamp of illness is soon gained."

CHAPTER SIX

The Enumeration of Metaphors

Then Sage Rigpé Yeshé spoke these words: "O great sage, listen! About the roots of (1) the condition [of the body], (2) diagnosis and (3) healing are coiled the nine trunks of (a) the properly functioning [body], (b) the malfunctioning [body], (c) visual examination, (d) feeling [the pulse], (e) questioning, (f) food, (g) behaviour, (h) medicine and (i) external treatment.

"The 47 branches [of these trunks] are as follows: of [the first trunk, i.e. the properly functioning] body, are (1) the humours, (2) the bodily constituents and (3) the impurities; of [the second trunk, i.e. the] malfunctioning [body], are (4) the causes. (5) the contributing conditions, (6) the entrances, (7) the locations [of the three humours], (8) the pathways, (9) the time of the arising [of illnesses], (10) [the situations of which the] result [is certain death], (11) reaction-imbalances and (12) the categories [of heat and cold disorders]; of [the third trunk of] visual examination are (13) the tongue and (14) the urine; of [the fourth trunk of examination through] feeling the pulse are three branches [including the pulse when there is (15) a wind disorder, (16) a bile disorder and (17) a phlegm disorder]; of [the fifth trunk of] questioning are (18) the conditions contributing to the arising [of the illness], (19) the symptoms and (20) foods and environment; of [the sixth trunk of] food are the six branches of food and drink [including (21) food and (22) drink for a person with a wind disorder, (23) food and (24) drink for a person with a bile disorder and (25) food and (26) drink for a person with a phlegm disorder]; of [the seventh trunk of] behaviour are the branches [of recommended behaviour for a person with a disorder of (27) wind, (28) bile and (29) phlegm]; of [the eighth trunk of] medicine are the three pairs of [branches representing] the tastes and inherent qualities [of medicines given for disorders of (30 & 31) wind, (32 & 33) bile and (34 & 35) phlegm], the six kinds of pacification [involving (36) liquid medicines and (37) medicinal oils for wind disorders, (38) decoctions and (39) powdered medicines for bile disorders and (40) pills and (41) tres sam for phlegm disorders] and the three kinds of cleansing [involving the use of (42) enemas, (43) purgation and (44) inducing vomiting]; of [the ninth trunk of] medical treatment are the three branches [for disorders of (45) wind, (46) bile and (47) phlegm].

"There are 25 leaves on the first [trunk], 63 on [the second trunk, i.e.] the malfunctioning [body], six on [the trunk of] visual examination, three on [trunk of] feeling the pulse and 29 on [the trunk of] questioning. [On the trunk of food there are] 14 for wind disorders, 12 for bile disorders and nine for phlegm disorders. There are six on [the trunk of] behaviour, and [on the trunk of medicine are individual leaves for] the nine tastes and nine inherent qualities of medicines, three liquid medicines, five kinds of medicinal oils, four kinds of decoctions, four powdered medicines, two kinds of pills, five kinds of tres sam and nine different remedies. [There are individual leaves for] the seven groups of medical treatment [on the ninth trunk]. Thus there are 88 for the basis of illness, 38 for diagnosis and 98 for the methods of healing. These all total 224.

"[On the first trunk] bloom the flowers of long life and freedom from illness and ripen the three fruits of Dharma [the teachings of the Awakened Ones], wealth and happiness. [These are the three fruits attained by the physician].

"This Root Tantra, in which is compiled the essential enumeration [of the branches of the science of healing], illustrated with metaphors, can be fully comprehended by those of keen intelligence, but not by those with dull minds. [The latter] should look to more elaborate texts."

Having spoken thus, Sage Rigpé Yeshé disappeared into the heart of the Sovereign Healer.

PART TWO

The Explanatory Tantra

CHAPTER ONE

Synthesis of the Explanatory Tantra

Then the Master, the all-surpassing, fully-endowed conqueror and physician, the King of Aquamarine Light and supreme benefactor, arose from that meditation and entered the meditation of healing called `The Lion of Speech'. As soon as he entered meditation, thousands of rays of multi-coloured light spread forth from the crown of his head in all the 10 directions, clearing away the physical defilements of all animate beings of the 10 directions and pacifying all illnesses of wind, bile and phlegm. Then upon drawing them [the light rays] back to the crown of his head, the illusory form of the Master named Sage Rigpé Yeshé emanated from his body and appeared in the sky before him.

> The physical defilements which were dispelled by the light rays refer to the three unwholesome physical acts of killing, stealing and sexual misconduct. As soon as the light rays returned to the crown of his head, there emerged from it one having the nature of Buddha's perfectly pure realization of the ultimate nature of the world, or the All-Appearing One, known by the name of Sage Rigpé Yeshé.

The manifestation of [Buddha's] speech named Sage Yilé Kyé prostrated before the Master and circumambulated him. Then he spoke: "O Master, Sage Rigpé Yeshé, thus you have delivered the Root Tantra, in which the main points are synthesized. How may we learn the Explanatory Tantra? May the physician, the Sovereign Healer, explain!" In reply to the request, the emanation of [Buddha's] body, Sage Rigpé Yeshé, said: "O great Sage Yilé Kyé: secondly, learning the Explanatory Tantra [involves the following]. In order for there to be freedom from illness, healing of illness, longevity, Dharma, wealth and happiness with regard to the body of man, who is chief of the six types of animate beings [the others being denizens of hell, spirits, animals, demi-gods and gods], I shall synthesize the main points of the science of healing. There are said to be four classifications of (1) the subject to be healed, (2) the healing agent, (3) healing methods and (4) the healer. [I shall] first teach the subject to be healed. In regard to what is involved in the healing?—(1) the body. What is healed?—(2) the illnesses that arise from it. The remedies which heal unbalanced humours are (3) behaviour, (4) food, (5) medicine and (6) external medical treatment. These remedies heal the humours [by giving] (7) long life and freedom from illness and (8) correction of physical imbalances. Towards this end there are three divisions of (9) methods of diagnosis, (10) methods of healing after [the nature of the disorder] has been understood and (11) the one who makes use of the methods of healing.

"Thus, O healer, the four roots and 11 branches are the synthesis of the Explanatory Tantra."

CHAPTER TWO

The Manner of Formation of the Body

Then Sage Yilé Kyé asked the Master, Sage Rigpé Yeshé : "O Master, Sage Rigpé Yeshé, how may we learn about the body which is formed [of the five elements]? We request the physician, the Sovereign Healer, to explain." The Master replied: "O great sage, listen! First, the teaching concerning the body formed [of the five elements], with respect to which there is healing, has the following seven divisions: (I) the manner of formation, (II) similes, (III) anatomy, (IV) characteristics [of the functions of the various parts of the body], (V) classifications, (VI) actions and (VII) the signs of death.

(I) THE MANNER OF FORMATION

"The teaching on the first, the manner of formation, has three parts: (A) the causes of formation, (B) the conditions contributing to growth and (C) the signs of birth.

(A) THE CAUSES OF FORMATION

"First, the causes of formation [of the foetus] in the womb are: non-defective sperm and blood of the father and mother, the consciousness [of the being who is about to enter the mother's womb] that is impelled by karma (i.e. a relation in a former life between this being and the man and woman by whom his next body will be conceived], mental distortions, and then the collection of the five elements.

> If this being has the karma to take birth as a male, he experiences hatred for his father and lust for his mother just prior to entering the sperm-blood mixture. If the being has the karma to be born a female, these passions are reversed.

For example, this is like the arising of fire from rubbing pieces of wood together.

Or the mother's blood may be likened to a flint, the

father's sperm to the iron, the consciousness that enters the mixture to a piece of bark and the embryo to the fire.

"If any of the following defects are present, [the sperm and blood are] not able to become the seed [of an embryo]. A wind disorder makes the sperm and blood coarse, dark and thick; a bile disorder makes them sour, yellow and foul-smelling; a phlegm disorder makes them light in colour, sticky, sweet and cool; a blood disorder makes them putrid; a wind and phlegm disorder makes them runny; a blood and bile disorder makes them pus-like; a phlegm and bile disorder makes them dark like sooty water; a wind and bile disorder makes them dry; a disorder of wind, bile and phlegm makes them [foul-smelling] like excrement and urine.

"If the [appropriate karma is not present, the consciousness does not enter [the sperm-blood mixture]. Without the earth element there is no formation; without the water element there can be no conglomeration [of the embryo or the sperm and blood]; without the fire element there is no maturation; without the wind element there is no growth; and without the space element there is no room for growth.

"Non-defective [regenerative fluid] which causes formation [of the foetus] in the womb [is as follows]. The sperm is white, heavy, sweet and abundant, and the blood is like liquid paint or hare's blood and can be easily washed [e.g. out of clothes].

"From the time a woman is of the age of 12 to 50, for three days [each month] wind opens the door of her womb and dark, odourless blood from the chyle which accumulates each month [in the vesicle of regenerative nutriment] falls from two large vessels. In a woman having her period, the signs of desire for men are shyness, facial ugliness [e.g. bagginess of the skin] and unsteady movement of the breasts, hips, neck, eyes and the sides of the body.

"[If there is sexual intercourse] during the first three days [of the menstrual period] or on the 11th of the 12 days following the menstrual period, a boy will not be conceived. [If there is intercourse] on the first, third, fifth, seventh or ninth day [of this 12-day period], a boy will be conceived; and on the second, fourth, sixth, eighth [10th or 12th] day, a girl will be conceived. The end of these 12 days is like the closing of a lotus, and thereafter the sperm is not held in the womb.

"If the sperm is more abundant, a boy will be born, but if the blood is more abundant, a girl will be born. If these are in equal quantities, a hermaphrodite or neuter will be born. [If the wind] acts [upon the blood-sperm mixture such that it separates into two or more globules] twins will be born.

"Birth with an inhuman form [e.g. that of some animal]and deformities occur due to impurities of harmful [wind, etc. acting upon the sperm or blood].

"Signs of conception, i.e. when the seed [i.e. both the male and female regenerative fluids] has been held [in the womb], are that the desire [of the women] is satisfied and [her] body feels exhausted and heavy.

> At the time of conception, the consciousness of those who have reached such a high spiritual attainment that they are able to choose their next birth enters the father's mouth and goes down through his sexual organ to the mother's womb. It seems to such a person that he is then entering a palace or mounting a throne. To others who have stored great merit in previous lifetimes, it seems that they are entering a lovely house. But to those who have much evil karma, it seems like entering a small hole in the ground or a dark cave from which there is no escape.

"The father's sperm forms the bones, brain and spinal cord, and the mother's blood forms the flesh, blood, solid organs and hollow organs. The [five] sense consciousnesses arise from one's own mind [i.e. the mind of the being who enters the mother's womb]. The flesh, bones, organ of smelling and odours are formed from the earth element. The blood, organ of taste, tastes and the moisture [in the body] arise from the water element. The warmth, clear colouration, the organ of sight and form are formed from the fire element. The breath, organ of touch and physical sensations are formed from the wind element. The cavities in the body, the organ of hearing and sounds are formed from the space element.

"In accordance with the actions to which one has been accustomed [in former lives, i.e. the kind of mental imprints one has stored from previous actions], appearances arise as one enters [the sperm-blood mixture]. Due to the collection and inter-relationship between these causes and conditions, the body is formed.

(B) THE CONDITIONS CONTRIBUTING TO GROWTH

"The teaching on the manner of growth after conception [is as follows:] the cause of growth of the embryo is [its] nucleus. On the right and left sides of the womb are two vessels which connect this nucleus with the vesicle of regenerative nutriment, which is its source of nourishment.

> First one vessel, the umbilical cord, arises from the nucleus of the foetus. It then splits in two, and the two branches join again in the vesicle of regenerative nutriment, which is the storage place for the chyle which goes to the foetus.

"Thus the chyle from the mother's food gradually causes the foetus to grow. For example, this is like water in a storage tank causing the fields to flourish.

"Further, for 38 weeks, [the foetus] goes through transformations due to the wind element and grows for nine months. During the first week of the first month, the mixture of sperm and blood is like a sour ferment that has been poured into milk [to make curd]. [During this first week, the regenerative fluids are transformed by the life-supporting wind.]

"During the second week, [the mixture] begins to [thicken and] become elongated.

> This thickening occurs due to the all-gathering wind, which is one of the pervasive winds that arise from the life-supporting wind.

"During the third week, it appears like curd.

> This transformation is caused by the karmic wind of action, which also arises from the life-supporting wind.

"There are methods which may be employed at this time by those desiring a boy, and they should be used before the sex [of the foetus] is clearly determined. With the influence of these [methods], the karma [of the foetus] may be [temporarily] overpowered [i.e. even if the foetus has the karma to become a girl, these methods can block the effects of this karma for this lifetime.] On [a day when the influence of the] star Victory [is strong on earth], form a statue of a boy from various kinds of iron and heat it over live coals until it is red-hot. [It should then be immersed] in milk or such ingredients as brown sugar or honey, and two handfuls of this liquid should be given [to the mother for her to drink]. The 'nutriment of the sun and moon' [referring to the kind of medicine called lhang tsher dmar po and mercury, respectively] is to be eaten [by the mother].

The mercury is prepared in a special way to remove its poisonousness, then it is mixed in equal quantities with the lhang tsher dmar po.

"And one should employ the omens of tying and fastening.

The former involves the following: wool is sheared from a male sheep and spun into thread by a good, healthy, young adolescent boy. Then three strands of this thread are strung together with knots tied in them, and the pregnant woman ties this around her abdomen with the knots over the womb. The second method involves fastening the statue of a boy against her womb with its head up.

"For eight months, [the pregnant woman] should avoid sexual intercourse, violent action, not sleeping at night, sleeping in the afternoon, forcefully tightening the abdominal muscles [either while defecating, urinating or for any other reason], hot acrid or heavy [foods], anything [such as food or medicine] that causes constipation, purgatives, medicine that induces vomiting, enemas or any medical treatment that causes a loss of blood [such as surgery or blood-letting]. Avoid these, for they will kill the foetus, and nothing more than a little blood will emerge from the womb [if the foetus is killed in the early stages of its growth].

"During the fourth [week], the foetus has either a round, a bisectional or an elongated form. From this a boy, a neuter [a hermaphrodite, or twins] or a girl will [correspondingly] gradually develop.

"Signs [of pregnancy] are heaviness of the hips, a feeling as if the body is charged with electricity, lack of appetite, yawning, stretching, lack of desire to move about or work, enlargement of breasts, attraction for sour foods and a variety of desires [especially for different foods] coming to mind [due to the karma of the child in her womb]. If [these desires] are blocked, the foetus will die or else have an unpleasing form, so even if they are harmful a little [of the desired food] should be mixed [with wholesome food] and given [to the mother] for the benefit [of both mother and child].

"During the fifth week, the second month, the first central [channel] in the body of the foetus forms, [called the 'vital channel'].

At this time its width is about that of a hair, and it is about half an inch long. It is situated behind the heart and is the basis, or the abode, of the mind. All the other channels gradually form from it. Along with the vital channel its two subsidiary channels form, one containing dark blood and the other, light blood.

"During the sixth [week], in reliance upon the nucleus [or elementary vital channel], the vital channel grows [to a length of 16 infant-sized fingerbreadths].

Four subsidiary channels form around it, encircling it like vines around a post, thus constricting the flow of wind through the vital channel, also called the 'central channel'. During this period, the form of the child is like that of a fish.

"During the seventh [week], the organ of sight takes form [i.e. the two channels for these organs appear].

Also at this time, many subsidiary channels arise from the vital channel at the throat, or 14 fingerbreadths up from the heart, and many others form on the crown of the head, or 16 fingerbreadths up from the throat. It should be noted that a fingerbreadth with reference to an infant's body means an infant's fingerbreadth, with reference to a child's body, a child's fingerbreadth, and so forth. During this week, many subsidiary channels also form in the region where the genitals will appear. Each of these channel centres at the throat, crown of the head and at the genital region is in the shape of an extended umbrella with the vital channel in the centre and the subsidiary channels branching out from it.

"During the eighth [week], in reliance [on the channel centre at the crown of the head], the shape of the head appears.

"During the ninth [week], the [general] shape of the upper and lower parts of the body forms.

"During the 10th [week], third month, the protrusions of the two shoulders and hips appears.

"During the 11th [week], the [general] form of the nine entrances to the body appears.

"During the 12th, the [general] form of the five solid organs appears.

"During the 13th, the [general] form of the six hollow organs appears.

"During the 14th [week,] the fourth month, the shape of the four limbs appears.

"During the 15th, the forearms and calves appear.

"During the 16th, the 20 toes and fingers appear. [The foetus now has a shape like that of a tortoise.]

"During the 17th, all the channels which connect the outer and inner body appear [e.g, the vessels lying just beneath the skin are related to the channels for the internal organs. At this point, the form of the body is complete.]

"During the 18th week, the fifth month, the flesh and fat form. [Previously they were not separate.]

"During the 19th, the major and minor ligaments form.

"During the 20th, the bones and marrow form.

"During the 21st, the outer skin covers [the body].

"During the 22nd week, the sixth month, the actual openings of the nine bodily entrances appear.

"During the 23rd, the head and body hair and the fingernails grow.

"During the 24th, the solid and hollow organs clearly mature [and begin to function]. At that time, [the foetus] begins to experience pleasure and pain.

"During the 25th, the movement of the wind [i.e. the breath] commences.

"During the 26th, the memory becomes clear.

> At this time, the infant remembers the act in one of his former lives that led to his present situation. With this insight he recognizes the nature of the round of existence and thereby has a feeling of sadness and a sense of renunciation.

"Then during the seventh month, from the 27th to the 30th week, all [the parts of the body] come to a clear state of completion.

"During the eighth month, from the 31st to the 35th week, all [the parts of the body] grow in size, and the mother and child alternate in turn with respect to their appearance.

> Sometimes most of the nutriment from the mother's food goes to the child, and as the result the mother's appear-

ance suffers and the child flourishes. At other times, the opposite is the case. During this period, if most of the nutriment steadily goes to the mother, the child may be born prematurely.

"During the ninth month, from the 36th week on, [the child recognizes his unclean surroundings and feels] disgust and unhappiness [and wishes to be in a more pleasant environment. By this time, he has lost his former clarity of memory.]

"[At the end of] the 37th [week], perverse thoughts arise [i.e. if the child is a boy, he feels hatred for his father and lust for his mother, and if a girl, the reversed passions arise].

"[At the beginning of] the 38th week [directly after the former passions have arisen, the child] turns over with his head down and emerges from the womb.

"However, [the period of gestation] takes longer if (1) [the foetus] is unable to develop due to [the mother's] losing blood [during pregnancy], (2) the womb grows very large [due to the mother eating much highly nutritious food], thus making birth difficult when the period of normal gestation is completed, or (3) [the mother's upward-moving] wind blocks the vagina [so that the foetus may not emerge].

Some pregnancies last 11 or 12 months and on rare occasions may last even more than a year due to the karma of the mother and child. In the sutras it is recorded that the son of King Dhöndhub remained in the womb for six years.

(C) The Signs of Birth

"When [the foetus] has thus grown and matured in the womb and nine months have passed, the time of birth is at hand. A boy will be born if (1) the [mother's] right hip is higher [and larger than the left].,(2) [her] body feels light, (3) [she] sees men in her dreams, or (4) [her] right breast enlarges first. Signs that a girl will be born are (1) [the mother's] desire to meet with men, (2) attraction for song, dance and jewellery, and (3) the opposite of the above [e.g. the left hip is higher and the left breast enlarges first]. If there is a mixture of these [signs], a neuter [or hermaphrodite] will be born, and if the centre [of the mother's abdomen is depressed and the sides are extended, twins will be born.

"Then the signs that birth is close at hand are (1) bodily

fatigue, (2) relaxing of the vulva, (3) heaviness of the lower part of body, (4) fluctuating pain in the hips, pelvic bones and lower abdominal region and itching of the genitals, and (5) heaviness [of the genitals]. [Then] the vulva opens naturally, much urine [is discharged], and pain arises. The woman about to give birth should have the needed auxiliaries and help at hand. [These will] greatly relieve the pain which will otherwise make her feel she is going to die [while giving birth].

CHAPTER THREE

Similes for the Body

In this chapter many similes are made, comparing the parts of the body to articles in an ancient Indian or Tibetan house. As these articles are not found in modern-day houses and are difficult to describe and, further, since this chapter is not of great importance, it will not be translated here.

CHAPTER FOUR

The Anatomy of the Body

Then Sage Rigpé Yeshé spoke these words: "O great sage, listen! These are four parts to the teaching on the anatomy of the body: (I) the teaching on the anatomy with regard to the quantities of the bodily constituents, (II) the teaching on the anatomy of the circulatory system, (III) the teaching on the anatomy of the vital areas with which there is danger [if they are seriously damaged] and (IV) the teaching on the anatomy of the cavities or passageways [in the body].

(I) ANATOMY— QUANTITIES OF BODILY CONSTITUENTS

"First, the quantity of wind [in an adult body] would fill the capacity of the urine bladder. The quantity of bile would fill the capacity of the scrotum, and the quantity of phlegm would fill three double handfuls. The quantities of blood and plasma would each fill seven double handfuls. The quantities of urine [as well as the fluid in the kidneys which will become urine] and lymph would each fill four double handfuls. The quantities of fat and body oil would each fill two double handfuls. The quantities of male and female regenerative fluids would each fill one handful. The quantity of brain matter would fill one double handful. The quantity of flesh is 500 fist-sizes, but for women there are 20 more due to their hips [an extra 10 fist-sizes] and breasts [also 10 fist-sizes]. With regard to the bones: there are 23 types as well as the 28 vertebrae in the vertebral column [not counting the large one at the top or the three small ones down at the base], 24 ribs, 32 teeth, 360 separate bones, 12 kinds of large joints and 210 small joints. There are 16 large and 900 small ligaments. There are 21,000 hairs [on the head] and [3.5] tens of millions of pores. There are five solid and six hollow organs and nine entrances. The [perfect] body of a person on earth is six feet square [from the feet to the head and from the fingertips of one outstretched arm to the fingertips of the other], but poorly formed bodies are three and one-half cubits [in length, or a little over five feet].

(II) ANATOMY — CIRCULATORY SYSTEM

"The teaching on the anatomy of the circulatory system [concerns] the four types of channels: (A) the channels of formation, (B) the channels of existence, (C) the channels of connections and (D) the channels of life:

(A) THE CHANNELS OF FORMATION

"There are three channels of formation that branch out from the heart. One of them goes upwards and thus the brain is formed. Ignorance [or mental dullness] relies upon and is located in the brain, and from it arise phlegm [disorders], which are located in the upper body. One of the channels [which is thick and only a few inches long] goes along the middle [of the body by the heart], and thus the vital channel is formed. Anger [arises in] dependence upon it and is located in the vital channel and the blood. Bile [disorders] arise from and are located in the middle body. One of the channels reaches down and thus the genitals are formed. Lust is located in the male and female genitals, and from it arise wind [disorders], which are located in the lower body.

(B) THE CHANNELS OF EXISTENCE

"There are four types of channels of existence [classified with respect to their functions]. Five hundred channels surround the channel of existence at the brain, and it is this channel that causes the sense organs to function. Five hundred channels surround the channel of existence at the heart [i.e. the vital channel], and it is this channel that brings about mental clarity [and a sense of identity]. Five hundred channels surround the channel of existence at the navel, and it is this channel that forms the body [from the beginning, when there is only the sperm-blood mixture, until there is a fully-grown body]. Five hundred channels surround the channel of existence at the genitals, and it is this channel that causes one's lineage of [male and female] children to increase. [These channels connect the areas] above, below and near [their respective centres and thus] hold together the entire body.

(C) THE CHANNELS OF CONNECTION

"There are two channels of connections—light and dark. Twenty-four large channels which increase the flesh and blood reach up in the manner of branches off the trunk-like vital channel [which is the dark channel on the right side of the body, also referred to as the roma].

The vital channel is dark because the blood, bile and heat are slightly stronger in it. The channel on the left side of the body, called the kyang-ma, is lighter in colour due to its greater content of phlegm and wind, but the difference again is slight. The vital channel contains little wind, and it reaches up next to the spinal column from the 13th vertebra from the top up to the base of the throat.

"Eight large hidden channels [hidden because they are deep inside the body] are connected to the internal solid and hollow organs. Sixteen manifest [i.e. they can be detected from outside the body] channels connect the outer limbs. Seventy-seven channels from which blood may be taken branch off from there.

"There are 112 principal channels with which there is danger [if they are damaged], and 189 minor channels which branch off [from them]. From these there branch off 320 minor channels in the outer, middle and inner [parts of the body], and 360 minor channels branch off from them. Seven hundred minor channels branch off from these, and from these there is a network of minor channels connecting the [entire] body.

"There are 19 small ligaments with their [individual] functions which reach down like roots from the 'ocean' of channels at the brain. Furthermore, there are 13 hidden channels which reach down like tassels [from the brain] to the solid and hollow organs. There are six major ligaments which are externally evident and which connect the limbs.

Actually there are only two, which are outwardly evident in three places: at the back of the neck, on both sides of the spine directly above the hips and above the heels.

"From these branch off 16 small ligaments [as well as many others still smaller].

(D) The Channels of Life

"Human beings have three [types of] channels of life. One [type] pervades the head and the entire body. One accompanies the movement of the breath.

These include the two air passageways from the nostrils to the lungs. Humans breathe in and out 21,600 times during each day and night. From these, 16,460 breaths contain wind of mental distortions, and for their duration, the mind is in an unwholesome attitude. The breaths containing wind of transcending awareness number 675, and for their duration, one experiences happiness and a wholesome frame of mind.

"One is like the reliance of life and ranges [over the entire body]. Because these [three types of channels] connect the inner and outer body and the entrances by acting as passageways for the wind and blood, thus enabling the body to grow and thrive, and because the life force resides in them, they are called '[vital] channels'.

(III) ANATOMY — VITAL AREAS

"The seven critical points are the flesh, fat, bones, ligaments, solid organs, hollow organs and channels. [Injury of] the flesh results in swelling; [injury of] the bones gives much pain; [injury of] the ligaments results in lameness; and [injury of] the channels, fat [especially that which covers the liver], solid or hollow organs results in loss of life. These are called 'critical' because [injury of them] is difficult to heal and [may] lead to death.

"There are 45 critical points of flesh, eight of fat, 32 of bone, 14 of ligaments, 13 of the solid and hollow organs and 190 of channels. [Among these] 62 are in the head, 33 in the neck, 95 in the upper and lower trunk and 112 in the four limbs. The number of critical points totals 320. From among these 96 are extremely critical. Once these are damaged, death is certain, for there is no cure even if [the physician is] skilled. Forty-nine points are said to be of medium criticalness, and these can be cured by the skilled. Although the remaining are described as critical, they are not said to be dangerous, for all [physicians] are able to heal them.

(IV) ANATOMY — CAVITIES OF PASSAGEWAYS

"There are both external and internal openings which act as pathways. The internal openings are the vital channel, bodily constituents and [openings for] the impurities.

The vital channel here refers to the second type of channel of life, i.e. the passageways for the breath. The bodily constituents refer specifically to the pathway of the chyle as it passes from the stomach to the various parts of the body. The progression is as follows: from the stomach to the liver, then to the blood, then to the flesh, from the flesh to the fat and then to the bone, from the bone to the marrow and finally to the regenerative nutriment, which is stored in the vesicle of regenerative nutriment. There are three kinds of openings for urine, excrement and perspiration.

"There are 13 pathways for the impurities and food [or chyle]. There are seven external openings in the head and two at the genital region. Women have the extra openings of the vulva and the breasts. Some channels are round, some thick, some narrow, some long and they are connected like the veins on the back of a leaf. Disorders [of wind, bile and phlegm] are caused by injuring the [internal] pathways by improper diet and behaviour, and they increase the chyle [as well as the other bodily constituents, impurities and the vital channel]. [When one of the humours] increases, it blocks [the passageways], and movement of the other two [humours] is disturbed. Unharmed, the openings are clear and there is happiness."

CHAPTER FIVE

Characteristics of the Body

Then Sage Rigpé Yeshé spoke thèse words: "O great sage, listen! The characteristics of the body are of two kinds: (I) the areas that are the objects of harm and (II) the humours, which are inflicters of harm. Due to the mutual interdependence of the humours, bodily constituents and impurities, [the body is] formed, thrives and is destroyed. Because [the aggregates compounded by these substances] are the root of [this process, they are called] the body.

(I) AREAS — OBJECTS OF HARM

"Firstly, among the divisions of the areas that are objects of harm, there are the digestive heat, the manner in which [it] transforms [the objects that are harmed], and the time of the completion of [their] results. The two divisions of the objects of harm are the bodily constituents and the impurities. The seven bodily constituents include the chyle, blood, flesh, fat, bone, marrow and regenerative fluid. The impurities are the excrement, urine, perspiration, etc. These too [are objects of harm]. The chyle increases the objects of harm [especially the blood]; the blood moistens [the body] and sustains life; the flesh covers [the body]; the fat lubricates it; the bones give it support; the marrow is transformed into essential nutriment; and the regenerative fluid brings about conception in the womb. The excrement [in the intestines] and the urine [in the urinary bladder] support [the organs and substances located above them while they are] decomposing. [Then they are] expelled [from the body]. The perspiration keeps the skin flexible and the pores firm.

"'Bodily heat' is the basis of digestion and refers to the bile that causes digestion. It is the warmth of all [three] humours, bodily constituents and impurities, and it gives freedom from illness, provides energy, a lively complexion and [long] life and increases the bodily constituents and the power of the bodily heat. [It differentiates the stomach contents into the wastes and chyle, then] causes [the former to leave] through the opening from the area of digestion. [Furthermore, it is] the constant door that [prevents undigested] food [from moving along] the path [of digested food]. If [the bodily heat] is strong, after digestion [the wastes] move downwards, but if it is weak, the food leaves [the body] still undigested. Bodily heat is the cause of food increasing the bodily constituents, a lively complexion and strength, for if the food is not digested, the chyle, etc. will not increase. If the bodily heat is protected by taking care to partake of warm food and drink and [following proper] behaviour [e.g. keeping the body warm], the strength and life of the body will thrive.

"The manner in which the bodily heat digests food [is as follows]: the life-supporting wind puts the food and drink into the stomach. The drink disintegrates [the stomach contents] and the oil [in the food] softens them. The fire-accompanying wind [in the lower region of the stomach] 'blows' upon the digestive bile [in the middle region of the stomach], which is like boiling medicine in the stomach.

> The simile here is that the action of the fire-accompanying wind upon the digestive bile and the stomach contents is like that of a fire blazing under a pot filled with medical ingredients. The digestive bile is stirred up by this and this makes for differentiation and separation of the stomach contents into wastes and chyle.

"First, mixing phlegm [in the upper region of the stomach] mixes together the food and drink of any of the six flavours that have been consumed. [During this process, the food and drink become] sweet and frothy, and [the power of] phlegm increases [throughout the body]. During the middle period [of digestion], the digestive bile digests [the stomach contents and they become] very hot and thus sour in taste, while the [power of] bile increases [throughout the body]. Finally, the fire-accompanying wind [in the lower region of the stomach] separates the chyle from the wastes, and [the stomach contents] become bitter, causing the [power of] wind to increase [throughout the body]. Due to the qualities of the food, which contain the five elements [earth, water, fire, air and space], the five elements of the body increase.

"The transformation process after the digested food has been separated into chyle and wastes [is as follows]: the wastes are separated into thick [solid] and thin [fluid] wastes in the intestines. The thick becomes excrement, and the thin becomes urine. The chyle is matured by the bodily heat of each of the bodily constituents. From the stomach it passes through the nine channels which receive chyle [and lead it] by way of the liver. In the liver it becomes blood; from blood [the superior nutriment] turns into flesh; from the flesh [the superior nutriment] turns into fat; from the fat it turns into bone; from the bone it turns into marrow; and from the marrow it turns into regenerative nutriment. The wastes [from] these [transformations turn into the following: the wastes, or inferior residue, from the chyle that goes to the liver turns into the mixing] phlegm in the stomach. [The inferior residue from the blood becomes] the bile in the gall bladder. [The inferior residue from the flesh turns into] the excretions from the cavities [of the eyes and ears]; [the inferior residue from the fat becomes] body oil [and perspiration]; [the inferior residue from the bones becomes] teeth, nails and body hair; [the inferior residue from the marrow becomes] skin, excrement and oil; [and the inferior residue from the regenerative nutriment goes down to the vesicle of regenerative nutriment and produces the] foetus. The bodily constituent of the regenerative nutriment has the finest colour [for it gives colour and strength to all the parts of the body], and although it stays in the heart [i.e. the vital channel, its power] pervades the entire body [like a light brightens a room]. It is the basis of life and produces a bright complexion and physical radiance.

"The duration for the completion of these products, i.e. the time it takes for the chyle from consumed food to turn into regenerative nutriment, is six days. But fertility medicine, etc. produces regenerative nutriment immediately [i.e. between five and six hours after consumption]. Most medicines do so [i.e. pass through the entire process of digestion, performing a particular function at each stage] in one 24-hour period.

(II) THE HUMOURS — INFLICTERS OF HARM

"There are eight [divisions in the explanation of the] humours, which are the inflicters of harm: (A) classification, (B) the process of conception, (C) nature, (D) bodily heat, (E) stomach, (vF) location, (G) functions and (H) characteristics.

(A) CLASSIFICATION

"There are three categories [of inflicters of harm]: wind, bile and phlegm. [Their] number and order are established from the point of view of their cause, nature, example and result. A body which is undisturbed thrives, but one which is disturbed is overcome.

"There are five kinds of wind: (1) life-supporting, (2) upward-moving, (3) pervasive, (4) fire-accompanying and (5) downward-clearing. There are five kinds of bile: (1) digestive, (2) colour-transforming, (3) accomplishing, (4) visually-operating and (5) complexion-clearing. There are five kinds of phlegm: (1) supportive, (2) mixing, (3) experiencing, (4) satisfying and (5) connecting.

(B) THE PROCESS OF CONCEPTION

"The explanation of the process of conception [with regard to the inflicters of harm is as follows]: in the first [moment] of conception, [they] are present in the semen and blood. This is, for example, like being formed from the poison of a poisonous insect [in that the three humours are the source of many physical ailments, yet they also contribute to the growth and development of the body].

(C) NATURE

"There are seven [physical] natures [which result from] an over-abundance [of any] of the humours due to diet or behaviour while the semen and blood are in the womb [i.e. during gestation]. If the wind [is predominant, the child's body will be] small; if the bile [is predominant, it will be] medium-sized; and if the phlegm [is predominant, it will be] large. It is best if [all three are of] equal strength and fair if [any of the] three pairs [i.e. wind and bile, bile and phlegm, or wind and phlegm are especially strong].

(D) BODILY HEAT

"There are likewise four types of bodily heat in the stomach. [Predominance of] wind [causes the bodily heat] to fluctuate; [predominance of] bile [makes it] sharp [or strong]; [predominance of] phlegm [makes it] weak; and [if all three humours are of] equal strength, it is balanced.

(E) STOMACH

"[Predominance of] wind [makes] the stomach [internally] firm [though not hard to the touch]. [This is characterized by a difficulty in defecating.] [Predominance of] bile [makes the stomach] loose [such that one must defecate frequently,] and [predominance of] phlegm [causes] the stomach to be middling [i.e. neither very firm nor loose].

(F) LOCATION

"Although [the three humours] are located throughout the body, they are [principally] found consecutively in (1) the region of the heart and below the navel [i.e. wind is located here], (2) [bile] between the heart and navel and (3) phlegm above the heart.

(G) FUNCTIONS

'The functions of the humours [are as follows]: wind exhales and inhales the breath, moves [the body], does [physical] work, expels [mucus, spittle and wastes], moves [through] the objects of harm [moving the blood through the vessels and keeping them clear], gives clarity to the sense organs [i.e. the five physical organs and the mind] and [by such means] sustains the body. The action of bile [results in] hunger and thirst, [upon which it] digests food, heightens bodily heat, clears complexion, courage and intelligence. Phlegm gives firmness to the body and mind, produces [desire for] sleep, connects the bone joints [acting as a lubricant], gives patience and lubricates the body, making it soft.

"In particular, the life-supporting wind is located at the crown of the head and moves along the throat and the breast-bone. It swallows food and drink, inhales, spits, sneezes, belches, gives clarity of mind and physical sense organs and holds the mind [together with the body]. The upward-moving wind is located in the region of the breast-bone and moves in the nose, the tongue and the throat. [Working in interaction with the life-supporting wind], it produces speech, and it also gives strength, [bodily] colour, energy and clarity of memory [and attention]. The pervasive wind is located in the heart [i.e. in the vital channel] and moves throughout the whole body. It lifts up and presses down, moves [the body] from one place to another, stretches out and draws in [the body, limbs, fingers and toes], opens and closes [the various bodily apertures] and is relied upon for most actions. The fire-accompanying wind is located in the stomach and moves through all the internal hollow organs [e.g. the intestines, gall bladder, channels in the heart, etc]. It digests food, separates the chyle from the wastes and gives nourishment to the objects of harm. The downward-clearing wind is located in the genital region and moves in the large intestine, the urinary bladder, the genitals and the thighs. It releases and retains semen, menstrual blood, excrement, urine and the foetus.

"The digestive bile is located [in the digestive tract] between [where the food is] not yet digested and [where it has been] digested. It digests food and [slightly] separates the wastes from the chyle, generates bodily heat, aids the other four [types of bile] and produces strength. The colour-transforming bile is located in the liver and transforms all the colours of the nutriment, etc. [i.e. the rest of the bodily constituents]. The accomplishing bile is located in the heart and contributes to self-confidence, pride, intelligence and the accomplishment of desires. The visually-operating bile is located in the eyes and gives the ability to see form. The complexion-clearing bile is located in the skin and gives the skin a clear complexion.

"The supportive phlegm is located along the breast-bone. It supports the other types of phlegm [e.g. it helps the mixing phlegm by holding up the food in the oesophagus so that it comes down slowly] and provides moisture [throughout the body, e.g. in the mouth]. The mixing phlegm is located [in the upper digestive tract where the food is] not yet digested, and it mixes together and decomposes the food and drink. The experiencing phlegm is located in the tongue and gives the ability to experience tastes. The satisfying phlegm is located in the head and satisfies the sense organs. The connecting phlegm is located in all the joints. It connects the joints and gives the ability to stretch out and retract [all the major and minor limbs].

(H) CHARACTERISTICS

"The characteristics of the humours, wind, bile and phlegm, [are as follows]: wind is characteristically rough, light, cold, subtle, hard and motile. Bile is characteristically oily, acrid, hot, light, bad-smelling and bears the quality of purging and moisture. Phlegm is characteristically cool and heavy, and acts as a softening agent, is gentle, firm and sticky."

CHAPTER SIX

The Actions and Classifications of the Body

Then Sage Rigpé Yeshé spoke these words: "O great sage, listen! The actions of the body are physical, verbal and mental and [fall into the categories of] wholesome, unwholesome and unspecified behaviour. In particular, the five senses apprehend their own objects.

"There are four classifications of the body with regard to: (A) sex, (B) age, (C) nature and (D) illness [or health].

(A) Sex

"There are three classifications in terms of sex: male, female and neuter [or hermaphrodite].

(B) Age

"The classifications of age [are as follows]: youth lasts until the age of 16. Then the bodily constituents, the [clarity of the] senses, complexion and strength increase, and middle-age lasts until the age of 70. Then old age lasts from then on, as [the clarity of the senses, etc.] decreases.

(C) Nature

"There are seven [types of human] natures [with regard to the three humours]: [a person whose nature is predominantly influenced by] just one [of the humours], [influenced by] a pair [of them] and [influenced by] all three equally.

"People who are influenced [predominantly] by wind have a stooped-over form, are thin and of dark complexion, talkative, unable to endure cold or wind, make a [rustling] sound when they move], have few [possessions and a short lifespan. They are light sleepers and have small bodies, they enjoy singing and laughing, fighting and archery, and they like sweet, sour and hot tastes. They have the qualities of a vulture, a raven and a fox.

"Those [influenced by the] nature of bile have great thirst and hunger, yellow hair and bodies, sharp minds and great pride. They perspire much and are bad-smelling, and they have a medium degree of wealth, lifespan and bodily size. They are fond of sweet, bitter, thick and cool foods, and they have the qualities of a tiger, a monkey and a fierce spirit.

"Those having the nature of phlegm have cool bodies, bone joints that do not protude, obesity, pale complexion, an erect posture and the ability to endure sustained hunger, thirst and [the pain of] mental distortions. They have large bodies, long life and much wealth. They are heavy sleepers, are slow to rise to anger, and they have kind natures. They are fond of hot, sour, thick and rough foods, and they bear the qualities of a lion and a buffalo [of a courageous and strong kind which goes before the herd as it goes out to graze in the morning and trails it as it returns in the evening in order to watch out for dangerous predators].

"[The nature of those who are predominantly influenced by] a pair or all [three of the humours] can be understood by combining [the above characteristics].

(D) Illness

"To classify with regard to illness, there are undisturbed and disturbed [bodies]. To be undisturbed is the normal state of the body, and one thus lives free of illness and has a long life. The body that has been overcome by illness is to be healed."

CHAPTER SEVEN

Signs of Death

Then Sage Rigpé Yeshé spoke these words: "O great sage, listen! There are four types of omens of death: (I) distant, (II) near, (III) uncertain and (IV) certain.

(I) DISTANT DEATH OMENS

"There are three types of distant signs: (A) the messenger [i.e. the person sent by the patient either to fetch a doctor or to bring him a sample of the patient's urine for analysis], (B) dreams and (C) character.

(A) Messenger

"A messenger who is remarkable [e.g. one in the guise of a yogi], a Buddhist monk or some similar person [e.g. one bearing a sense of dignity and inspiring faith in others] is a sign of the recovery of the patient. If the opposite is the case [e.g. if the messenger is a woman, a neuter, a cripple or comes riding a mule or a buffalo, recovery] will not occur. There will be no success [in the treatment] if the messenger [upon his arrival at the doctor's] is trembling with fright, panting, holding a stone or a fruitless branch; or if [on the way, he meets someone who] tells him of [bad news in a] faraway region; if [either on the way or upon his arrival], he commits an evil deed or [wears] inauspicious ornaments [e.g. a red flower, weapons or ornaments of the opposite sex]; or if he speaks [disparagingly upon his arrival]. [In such cases, there will be no recovery even if the messenger has the above favourable qualities]. It is a sign of death of the patient if the messenger arrives: when the doctor has coarse thoughts [or behaviour] or is speaking ignorantly [or improperly]; when there is cutting [of hair, wood, etc.] and destruction [e.g. of a house]; [when there is a performance of] a fire offering or a ritual which is enacted seven days after a person has died. It is bad if [the messenger] starts on his way on the 6th, [16th, 26th], 4th, [14th, 24th], 9th, [19 or 20th] days of the lunar month, the time of a solar or lunar eclipse, bad [influence of the] planets and stars, or at night. While [the messenger is] going [to the doctor's, or the doctor is on his way to the patient], it is a bad sign if: anything is cut or breaks on the way; one hears, hears of or sees weeping or a killing; a cat, monkey, otter or snake crosses one's path; or one sees anything unpleasant [e.g. a cripple, an accident or an evil deed]. Wholesome signs include seeing [or hearing] a wholesome act [e.g. the reading of a scripture or the performance of a religious offering], seeing a vessel full of grain or yoghurt, etc. [e.g. jewels or gold], a bell [used in religious ceremonies], a lamp or flowers [being used as a religious offering], fried rice, jam, an image of a divine being [e.g. a statue of Buddha], [a person wearing] white bodily ornaments, [someone involved in] spiritual practice, the raising of a banner [e.g. on top of a house], a flame burning, horses, sheep, cattle, etc. with their young, pleasant sounds, food, drink or ornaments. Either seeing such occurrences on the way [either to the patient or the doctor] or seeing them brought into someone's home is a wholesome indication that the patient will recover. [Seeing someone] take yoghurt or alcohol, etc. from his home, a fire dying when there is no wind, and the breaking of a vessel are bad omens.

(B) DREAMS

"Signs that one [i.e. the patient] has been seized by the Lord of Death [and, thus, is soon to die] are dreaming that one is riding a cat, monkey, tiger, fox or a corpse. Dreams of [oneself] riding naked to the south upon a buffalo, a horse, pig, donkey or a camel [indicate] death. Omens that one has come under the power of the Lord of Death are [dreaming of] a willow tree with a bird's nest [on top] growing from the crown of one's head, a palmyra tree or a thorny tree growing from the one's heart, lotuses emerging [from one's heart], falling off a cliff, sleeping in a cemetery, one's head breaking, being surrounded by crows or spirits of beasts that eat their young [e.g. scorpions], the skin falling from one's limbs, entering the womb of one's mother, being carried along by a river, being stuck in a swamp, being swallowed by a fish, receiving iron or gold, losing in trade or quarrel, wishing to dance, taking a bride, being naked, having one's hair and beard shaved, drinking alcohol with deceased acquaintances or being dragged by them [along the ground], wearing red clothes and garlands, and dancing with deceased acquaintances. Such dreams are not good, and a patient who continually has such dreams due to an ailment blocking the passage through which consciousness moves [i.e. the vital channel] will die. But a healthy person will not necessarily [die as a result of frequent dreams of this sort] for he may be freed of them through worship.

"The six kinds of [dreams of] (1) seeing, (2) hearing or (3) experiencing [something that was witnessed during waking hours], (4) praying [for some desired object], (5) fulfilling [one's desire] and (6) those arising from ailments, [as well as dreams in] the early part of the night and dreams that are forgotten do not have results.

> Dreams in the early part of the night may arise due to an obstruction of the vital channel by the mixing phlegm as it begins to digest food. In the middle of the night this channel may be blocked by the digestive bile, and late at night it may be obstructed by the fire-accompanying wind. Thus dreams at these times do not generally produce effects.

"If [a dream is] seen and clearly [remembered upon awakening, assuming that one awakens shortly after the dream has occurred, it does produce results. [At this time, if one dreams of meeting and worshipping] a deity, [or seeing] a great buffalo, [holy] men or famous men, a flame burning, an [overflowing] lake, blood and filth smeared on one's body, wearing white clothes, [raising] a banner or an umbrella, receiving fruit, climbing up a mountain, a fine house or a fruit-laden tree, riding a lion, an elephant, a horse or cow, crossing a river or ocean, going towards the northeast, escaping from misery [e.g. from a prison or a dark room], defeating one's enemies or being praised by a deity or one's parents, one will have long life, freedom from illness and gain wealth.

(C) Character

"The teaching on death omens [with regard to] changes in character of a normal person [i.e. anyone ill or healthy, is as follows]: [if for no reason] one hates one's doctor, medicine, spiritual guide or friends [although one previously felt love and respect for them, or vice versa] or for no reason one becomes virtuous, attractive in appearance, healthy or wealthy [when this was not the case previously], or vice versa, it is an omen of death. [The following situations are also omens of] death: always having poor bodily colour or unhappiness, crows not eating the offerings one has set out for them, water not remaining on one's chest but rather quickly drying after bathing, sound not being produced by knocking the finger-nails [of one hand against those of the other], becoming weaker [regardless of how much one] eats, a change in one's bodily odour, [finding oneself with many] lice or louse eggs [although previously one had few or none] or [finding that one has] none [although previously there were many]. A person [to whom any of the following situations occurs] is said to have come under the power of the Lord of Death: one's sensual desires become dull, one's temper changes from what it had been [e.g. a hot-tempered person for no apparent reason becomes very patient, or vice versa] or one's behavioural faults or virtues change from what they had been [for no apparent reason]. One will die if, when the sun is shining, [one cannot see one's shadow, one cannot see one's reflection in a] mirror or [smooth] water, or [when looking at the] sky, [one sees one's own] image with no head or limbs.

(II) NEAR DEATH OMEN

"Then there are two types of near omens [of death]: (A) near and (B) extremely near.

(A) Near

"With regard to near omens [of death], one will die [if any of the following situations occur]: blood emerges from any of the nine entrances [e.g. the mouth, nostrils, etc.] although one has not been poisoned or pierced by a weapon; immediately forgetting what has been said; retraction of the penis [leaving just] the scrotum hanging or vice versa [i.e. the testicles retracting, leaving the penis hanging]. [If any of the above omens occur in a person with normal health, he has approximately six months to live]. [Other near omens include:] a strange sound being produced when clearing the throat or sneezing, not detecting the odour of a lamp that has just burnt out, having no sensation if one's hair is pulled out, the appearance of oil on the crown of the head, new parts or swirls appearing in one's hair or eyebrows, lines [in the shape of] a new moon appearing on the forehead or around the lips, change in one's sensual perception without [apparent] reason, i.e. perceiving more or less [than previously], not seeing the form of one's wrist [while touching the fingers to the top of head], lack of lustre in the whites of the eyes like those of a sleeping rabbit, or the turning inward and loss of colour of the pupils. One will die if one's ears stick [to the sides of the head], the soft roar [heard when the palms are pressed to the ears] is cut, or if there is no shadow from the vapour [rising] from the head [due to the absence of perspiration on the head, even on hot days]. [Other signs of] death are the flaring of the nostrils and the appearance of [a film of] light mucus [below the nostrils], [darkening of the centre strip on the tongue, drying and shortening [of the tongue, resulting in an] inability to speak, the lower lip hanging down and the upper lip turning up, the face becoming blotchy, the breath cold and the teeth dark, the inhalation coming in gasps and the disappearance of [bodily] heat. [Other phenomena] which are explained as omens of death are a hot feeling while one's body [has a] cold ailment, [e.g.] casting off hot [clothing, etc.] although suffering from a cold ailment or, likewise, casting off [such things as] cool [towels, etc.] while suffering from a heat disorder, or no benefit being derived from the customary medication [e.g. cool medicine given for heat disorders], but finding that the opposite medication seems to help [e.g. hot medicine given for a heat disorder].

(B) Extremely Near

"[The signs of] extremely near death are the gradual fading of the [power of the] five elements [in the body] and the five sense organs. [First], due to the disappearance of the power of the earth element into the water element, form cannot be seen [clearly]. Due to the disappearance of the power of the water element into the fire element, the entrances [to the body] become dry. Due to the disappearance of the power of the fire element into the wind element, [bodily] heat diminishes, and due to the disappearance of the power of the wind element into the space element, the breath stops. Due to the diminishing of the eye organ, form is not [seen] clearly and disappears into sound. Due to the diminishing of the ear organ, sound is not [heard] clearly and disappears into smell. Due to the diminishing of the nose organ, smells are not [sensed] clearly and disappear into taste. Due to the diminishing of the tongue organ, tastes are not [experienced] clearly and disappear into physical contact. Due to the diminishing of the body organ, physical contact is not felt. [Finally all the senses disappear into the vital channel, and mental consciousness leaves the body].

(III) UNCERTAIN OMENS OF DEATH

"Uncertain omens of death. Although omens of death may appear due to many kinds of illness, the omens of death may be dispelled by dispelling the illness. However, if the omens remain firm even after [the illness] has been dispelled, death is certain.

(IV) CERTAIN OMENS OF DEATH

"[Certain omens of death.] A patient is certain to die if his external, internal and vital bodily constituents, i.e. his flesh, chyle and channels, malfunction. Even if one performs a variety of religious services in order to [dispel] the sickness, they are of no avail, for death is certain.

"Thus once the omens of death, which destroy the body, have disturbed the humours, bodily constituents and impurities, they destroy one another and life is lost. This is similar to the destruction of Mount Meru when the elements [earth, water, fire and air] are in a period of transformation. Ignorance of the omens of death prevents [knowing] when to give and when not to give treatment. By not knowing this, one fails to gain a good reputation. Therefore, those desiring to be wise understand the omens of death.

"One may reverse the omens [of death with regard to] dreams, character, distant and uncertain omens by collecting religious merit, reading [scriptures], meditating and reciting mantras for the three meditational deities. For near and certain omens, save the lives of animals that are destined to be killed. There are no methods for reversing extremely close omens."

CHAPTER EIGHT

The Causes of Illnesses

Then Sage Yilé Kyé asked: "O Master, Sage Rigpé Yeshé, how may one learn the principal of the rise and decline of illnesses ? May the physician, the Sovereign Healer, explain." The Master spoke: "O great sage, listen! The instructions concerning the principle of the rise and decline of illnesses which arise from the aggregates [of the body] which is to be cured is explained as having seven [parts]: (I) causes, (II) contributing conditions, (III) the manner of entrance [of illnesses], (IV) locations [of disorders of the three humours], (V) characteristics, (VI) classifications and (VII) individual subjects.

(I) CAUSES

(1) "First, there are two kinds of causes, (A) distant and (B) near.

(A) Distant Causes

"There are two [kinds of] distant causes: (1) general and (2) specific.

(1) General Causes

"For countless aeons the humours have been disturbed in a variety of ways, thus inflicting the body with pain. As it is not possible to teach the individual causes of each [disturbance], here is an explanation of the general cause of all illness. There is but one cause of all illness, and this is said to be ignorance due to not understanding the meaning of identitylessness. For example, even when a bird soars in the sky, it does not part from its shadow. [Likewise,] even when all creatures live and act with joy, because they have ignorance, it is impossible for them to be free of illness.

(2) Specific Causes

"Specific causes. The three [mental] poisons of desire, hatred and confusion arise from ignorance, and from these, the results of wind, bile and phlegm disorders are produced.

(B) Near Causes

"The near causes. Undisturbed wind, bile and phlegm are the causes of illness and when they are disturbed and in disequilibrium, they are of the nature of illness. [At such a time,] they harm the body and life and give suffering. Disturbance of bile burns the bodily constituents. Because it is hot, being of the nature of fire, although it remains in the lower portion of the body, it flames up to the higher. All ailments of heat, without exception, arise from it. Disturbance of phlegm smothers the heat of the body. It is heavy and cool, being of the nature of earth and water, and although it remains in the upper portion of the body, it falls to the lower. All ailments of cold, without exception, arise from it. Wind pervades both heat and cold. If it is with the sun [i.e. a heat ailment], it aids burning, and if with the moon [i.e. a cold ailment], it aids cooling. It moves throughout the upper and lower, inner and outer [regions of the body] and disturbs and causes to rise both [ailments of] heat and cold. Thus, wind is a cause of all ailments."

CHAPTER NINE

The Conditions Contributing to Illnesses

Then Sage Rigpé Yeshé spoke these words: "O great sage, listen! In addition to the causes, there are three kinds of contributing conditions which bring about [illness]: (A) formation-increasing conditions, (B) storing-arising conditions and (C) manifesting conditions. Because [the first] form and increase [illness], they are called 'formation-increasing'; because [the second] store and cause [illness] to arise, they are called 'storing-arising'; and [the third kind] are manifesting conditions because they cause stored [illness] to become manifest.

(A) Formation-increasing Conditions.

"Formation-increasing conditions of: (1) time, (2) sensory experience and (3) behaviour produce disorders when they are insufficient, excessive or perverse.

(1) *Time*

"There are three times—of heat, cold and rain. These are insufficient if there is little heat, cold or rain [during these seasons] and they are excessive if there is too much. They are perverse if there is no [heat, cold or rain during their proper seasons, e.g. if it is very cold during the hot season].

(2) *Sensory Experience*

"Insufficient [sensory experience] means little or no contact between the sense organs and their objects, and a great deal of the same is excessive contact. Perverse contact is said to be [sensory perception of] extremely close or distant, large or small, fearful or ugly objects.

(3) *Behaviour*

"Behaviour is of three [kinds]: physical, verbal and mental. Little or no action is insufficient. Very forceful action is excessive, and forcefully withholding or tightening [one's muscles when defecating, urinating or sneezing], twisting [one's body or limbs] and unwholesome acts are perverse action.

(B) STORING-ARISING CONDITIONS

"Storing, arising and pacification are the three [stages involved in a disturbance of any of the humours, and these are under the influence of] (1) causes, (2) nature [of the disturbance of the humours] and (3) time.

(1) Causes

"Rough qualities, etc. (i.e. other qualities of food, climate, etc. which contribute to wind disturbances] combined with warmth store [a potential] wind ailment, cold causes it to arise and oil and warmth pacify it. Likewise, acrid qualities, etc. combined with coolness store [a potential] bile ailment, heat causes it to arise and gentle qualities, etc. combined with coolness pacify it. Heavy and oily qualities combined with coolness store [a potential] phlegm ailment, warmth causes it to arise and rough qualities, etc., pacify it.

(2) Nature

"[Disturbances of each of the humours] are stored and increase in their own location [as described in the Root Tantra]. The causes of disturbances from the [above] causes [make one] desire contrasting qualities [e.g. oily qualities for a wind disorder]. [When a disorder of one of the humours] arises, it enters incorrect pathways [i.e. it moves from its own natural location to the location of the other humours and] shows its own symptoms.

(3) Time

"The three [seasons] of early summer and so forth [i.e. late summer and autumn] are the time of wind ailments.

> Early summer is the time they are stored, late summer— referring here to the time of monsoon—is the time they arise and autumn is the time of their pacification.

"[The corresponding times of] bile are late summer, [autumn and early winter, and those of] phlegm are late winter, [spring and early summer]. During the season of early summer, [potential disturbances of] wind are stored by light and rough qualities of habitat, physique, diet and behaviour, but due to the warmth they do not arise. Due to the rain, wind and cold of late summer, they arise, [then] in the autumn they are pacified due to conditions of oiliness and warmth. [Potential disturbances of] bile are stored in late summer due to oily conditions prevailing then, but due to the coolness they do not arise. They arise in autumn, with its qualities of oiliness and warmth, and are pacified by the coolness of early winter. The cool, oily, heavy qualities of late winter cause [potential disturbances of] phlegm to be stored, [but they are] concealed [by the cold] and thus do not arise. The warmth of the sun in spring causes them to arise, and the light and rough qualities of early summer pacify them.

(C) Manifesting Conditions

"However, even if the time of [their] appearance has not come, they may be caused immediately by [improper] diet and behaviour. There are, to be precise, two kinds of manifesting conditions: (1) general and (2) specific.

(1) General

"The conditions which generally cause all illnesses to become manifest are the seasons of their arising [as described above], spirits, poison, unhealthy diet, improper medication, and the fruition of negative actions.

(2) Specific

"The specific conditions that cause wind ailments to arise are: over-consumption of bitter, light and rough [food or medicine], exhaustion due to strong desire, lack of food and sleep, forceful physical and verbal activity on an empty stomach, much loss of blood, diarrhoea or vomiting, forcefully exhaling air [for a long time, especially air with the scent of camphor or sandalwood], weeping from exhaustion, grief, much mental or verbal activity, frequent consumption of unnutritious foods [or unripe fruits, grains, vegetables, etc.] and forcefully withholding or expelling [when defecating, urinating or sneezing].

"The conditions that cause the heat of bile [disorders] to become manifest are: over-consumption of hot, acrid, salty and oily [food or medicine], strong anger, sleeping in the afternoon when it is hot, then doing hard work immediately thereafter, carrying too heavy burdens, digging in hard soil, practising archery, wrestling, running, becoming fatigued due to moving about and working [during the heat of the day], being thrown by a horse, falling off a cliff, having earth cave in on oneself, being struck by rocks or sticks, and eating or drinking too much meat, butter, brown sugar or alcohol, etc.

"The conditions that cause the cold of phlegm [disorders] to become manifest are: over-consumption of bitter, sweet, heavy, cool and oily [food or medicine], relaxing after overeating, sleeping during the day or on a moist surface [e.g. wet grass], entering water and then becoming chilled due to wearing thin clothes, eating unripe or stale wheat or peas, goat meat, the flesh of thin cattle, rotten meat, fat, grain oil [including mustard, peanut and sunflower oil], butter, rotten food, all raw food such as raw unripe leaves [of pea plants, etc.], raw stale turnips and raw mountain garlic, uncooked or burnt food, [cold] leftovers, cold liquid goat's milk, curd, skimmed milk or tea, too much food and drink and eating again before the food [in one's stomach from the last meal] has been digested.

"Combinations of the above conditions lead to dual and triple disorders of the humours."

CHAPTER TEN

The Manner of Entrance of Illnesses

Then Sage Rigpé Yeshé spoke these words: "O great sage, listen! Thus the manner of entrance [of an illness] after [a disorder] has been produced by the [appropriate] causes and conditions [is as follows]: the four kinds of conditions [contributing to illness—time, spirits, food and behaviour—] shoot [the arrows of the three kinds of conditions—formation-increasing, storing-arising and manifesting—] at the target of the three humours. One of the targets is struck, and [the others are thereby] struck [as well] due to their inter-relationship.

"Furthermore, wind is located in the bones, bile in the blood and perspiration, and phlegm is located in the remaining [bodily constituents]. Thus the manner of their mutual dependence [is as follows]: a disturbance of the humours harms the bodily constituents, and both [disturbances] harm the impurities. Further, the nutriment of food that has characteristics similar to those of the cause of an illness is spread to all the [bodily] cavities by the pervasive wind. Then there is a malfunctioning in all of the cavities that the chyle reaches. At such a time, [illnesses] are stored and increased, each in their own location, by [contributing] behaviour. This is similar to the falling of rain when clouds gather in the sky. If a stored [illness] meets [the appropriate] conditions, it must certainly arise. Once it enters the six pathways [the skin, flesh, channels, bones, solid and hollow organs], there arise unhappiness and illness.

"The locations upon which [an illness] depends once it has entered [the body are as follows]: wind [ailments] are located in the lower stomach [intestines], ball joints of the hips, bones, [any place where there is] physical sensation, the ears, and especially in the lower stomach and the large intestine. Bile [ailments] are located at the navel, in the stomach, blood, perspiration, chyle, lymph, eyes, skin, and especially in the middle stomach. Phlegm [ailments] are located in the chest, throat, lungs, head, chyle, flesh, fat, marrow, regenerative fluid, excrement, urine, nose, tongue, and especially in the upper stomach."

CHAPTER ELEVEN

The Characteristics of Illnesses

Then Sage Rigpé Yeshé spoke these words: "O great sage, listen! There are three characteristics of illnesses: (I) increase, (II) decrease and (III) disturbance [of the humours, bodily constituents and impurities]. The causes and symptoms of an increase and decrease of the humours, bodily constituents and impurities will be explained.

"First, the causes of an increase or decrease of the humours are lack of desire for food and behaviour [that are good for one's constitution] and seeking [unwholesome food and activities]. [Another cause is] rejecting healthy activities and participating in unhealthy ones. These both result in the increase and decrease [of the humours].

"Second, the bodily heat [initially] resides in its own location, [the middle region of the stomach, but] some portion of it is located in all the bodily constituents. Its dwindling and flaring up cause an increase and decrease [in the bodily constituents].

Low digestive heat results in an increase of very low-quality chyle as one's food has not been well digested. A surplus of heat results in the drying up of the chyle and a corresponding decrease in the rest of the bodily constituents.

"[An increase or decrease in the] first [of the bodily constituents, i.e. the chyle] results in the increase and decrease of the following [bodily constituents in the digestive chain]. Know that the impurities [do not fall into imbalance of their own accord, but rather] are struck [by an imbalance of the humours and bodily constituents], which results [in their corresponding increase and decrease].

(I) INCREASE

"Symptoms [of increase]. The symptoms of an increase of wind are: dryness [of the body], dark complexion, attraction to warmth, trembling, bulging of the abdomen, constipation, talkativeness, dizziness and diminishing strength, sleep and [clarity of] the senses. Increase of bile causes yellowing of the stool, urine, skin and eyes, [great] hunger and thirst, over-heating of the body, little sleep and diarrhoea. Increase of phlegm causes diminishing bodily warmth, inability to digest food, bodily heaviness, light complexion, lassitude, looseness of the limbs, abundance of saliva and mucus, much sleep and difficulty in breathing. [The symptoms of] an increase of chyle are similar to those for phlegm. An increase of blood causes red itching spots on the skin, internal sores, ailments of the spleen, leprosy, knotty tumours on the skin, ailments of the blood and bile, yellowing of the eyes, ailments of the gums and palate, difficulty in moving, and reddening of the eyes, urine and skin. Increase of flesh causes goiter, protrusions of flesh on the skin, and abundance of flesh. Increase of fat causes lassitude and fattening of the breasts and paunch. Increase of bones leads to the growth of extra bones and teeth. Increase of marrow results in bodily heaviness, difficulty in focussing the eyes on an object, and thick bone joints. Increase of semen leads to [the formation of] stones [in the kidneys which are discharged through the urinary tract, causing much pain while urinating] and attraction to women. Increase of excrement causes bodily heaviness, bulging of the abdomen, and noise [and pain] in the intestines. Increase of urine causes pain at the tip of the penis and vulva and the feeling that one needs to urinate again immediately after having done so. Increase of perspiration results in an abundance of perspiration, unpleasant bodily odour, and skin ailments [e.g. itching]. Increase of the small substances [e.g. ear, wax, mucus, and water in the eyes] causes heaviness, violent itching or skin irritation and bodily odour.

(II) DECREASE

"[Symptoms of decrease]. Decrease of wind results in low energy, little speech, physical discomfort, unclear memory and attention, and the appearance of the symptoms of an increase of phlegm. Decrease of bile causes diminishing bodily warmth and colour, coldness and a dark complexion. Decrease of phlegm leads to a lack of phlegm in the places where it is normally located [i.e. four of the bodily constituents], dizziness, palpitation of the heart and a loosening of the joints. Decrease of chyle causes drying of the flesh, difficulty in swallowing food, roughness of the skin and illness which makes one unable to bear loud noise. Decrease of blood causes the vessels to become loose [i.e. soft due to lack of blood], roughness of the skin and [desire for] cool [sensual contact] and sour [foods]. Decrease of flesh results in pain in the joints [as if they were broken] and the joining of the bones with the skin [due to the lack of flesh between them]. Decrease of fat causes one to sleep little, drying of the flesh, and [one's complexion to] turn light blue. Decrease of bones leads to the falling out of the hair, teeth and nails. Decrease of marrow results in hollowness of the bones, dizziness and the forming of a film over the eyes. Decrease of regenerative fluid causes the appearance of blood [from the genital organs, and a male] feels that his scrotum is hot. Decrease of excrement causes sound to be emitted from the intestines [due to the movement of wind] and pain to be felt on the sides of the abdomen and at the heart due to the upward movement [of the wind]. Decrease of urine leads to a change in colour [of the urine] and difficulty in urinating, such that only a little is discharged. Decrease of perspiration causes cracking of the skin and makes the body hairs stand on end and fall out. Know that [a decrease of] the small substances results in their absence in their proper locations and the arising of chronic ailments. Since the bodily constituents depend upon the impurities, increase [of the latter] produces [illness], and [their] decrease is detrimental to the strength [of the bodily constituents]. Radiance [i.e. the finest of all the bodily constituents, which is the foundation of life and resides at the heart] decreases due to mental suffering, [resulting in] fear, emaciation, timidity, unhappiness and a diminishing lively complexion. Remedies [e.g. vitamins], milk and meat juice are the medicines [to be given to such a person].

(C) Disturbance

"[Symptoms of disturbance]. [Symptoms of a] wind [disturbance are]: resilience of the pulse [i.e. when the physician presses the vessels firmly, the pulse disappears, but when pressed lightly, it returns or 'bounces back'], urine that is clear like water and forms no sediment when left standing, desire to move about, forceful sighing, an unsteady, flighty mind, dizziness as if one were intoxicated, a humming and rustling sound in the ears, a tongue that is dry, red and rough, an astringent taste in the mouth, shooting pains that move [about the body], coldness, shivering, pain all over the body when one moves, lassitude, cramps in the limbs such that when they are outstretched they are difficult to retract, and when retracted difficult to stretch out, feeling as if [the flesh has] separated [from the skin and the bones have separated at their joints], feeling as if [one's bones are] broken, feeling as if [one's eyes and other organs are] bulging out, feeling as if [one's body has been] bound up, great pain when moving, sudden rising of body hair and goose bumps which quickly passes, insomnia, yawning, trembling, desire to stretch, hot temper, a feeling as if the hip bones and the base of the spine as well as all the other bones were being pounded, aching and shooting pains in the spinal, column from the base of the skull down to approximately two inches above the first vertebra, in the chest and the jaw bone, loosening of the sixth and seventh vertebrae and pain if they are pressed, dry heaves, the emission of soft, bubbly saliva from coughing at early dawn, abdominal noises, [and especially strong] pain in the evening and early dawn after one's food has been digested.

"Symptoms of a bile disturbance are a strong, 'finely twisted', fast pulse, orange, bad-smelling urine [from which there is] much vapour, headaches, heat of the flesh, [food tastes] sour and bitter, much [pale yellow] phlegm on the tongue [in the morning], dryness of the openings of the nostrils, an orange hue in the whites of the eyes, shooting pains in the region [of the bile disorder], little sleep at night but an inability to stay awake during the day, salty, orange mucus [coming up from the throat], great thirst, evacuation and vomiting of blood and bile, much perspiration, unpleasant body odour, orange complexion, and [the body becomes] soft and rotten. The illness is [strongest] at noon, midnight and while digesting food.

"Symptoms of a phlegm disturbance are a faint [such that it cannot be felt unless one's fingers are pressed hard against the vessels], weak, slow pulse, pale urine with little odour or vapour, inability to distinguish tastes, pale tongue, gums and palate, pale, swollen eyes [and cheeks], abundance of mucus in the nose and throat, a dazed feeling, physical and mental heaviness, poor appetite, lack of bodily warmth, weak digestion and little strength, pain in the kidneys and the base of the spine, swelling of the body, growth of goiter, vomiting and evacuation of food and phlegm, unclear awareness and memory, much sleep, lassitude, skin irritation, stiffness, tightness of the joints, gaining of weight, and procrastination. [Phlegm ailments] arise when the weather is moist, at twilight, in the early morning and immediately after eating.

"These symptoms of increase, decrease and disturbance that have been explained cover all illnesses. All combinations of disorders may be known from these symptoms, and it is impossible that there might be any symptoms of illness not included here."

CHAPTER TWELVE

The Classification of Illnesses

Then Sage Rigpé Yeshé spoke these words: "O great sage, listen! There are three classifications of illnesses: (I) with respect to the cause, (II) with respect to the type of patient and (III) with respect to the characteristics of the illness.

(I) WITH RESPECT TO THE CAUSE

"First, there are three classifications with respect to the cause: [ailments that arise due to] (A) the humours of this life, (B) from the actions committed in former [lifetimes] and (C) from a combination of the above two. The first [type of ailment] arises due to a collection of causes and conditions [causing an imbalance in humours]. [These are of three types: minor ailments, ailments caused by spirits and ailments arising due to an unwholesome action committed in the early part of one's present life]. Those [ailments] arising due to actions [committed during former lifetimes] rapidly worsen without [apparent] cause. [These can only be cured by religious practice in addition to medication.] [Ailments arising from a combination of the arising from a combination of the above two causes] rapidly worsen due to a minor [apparent] cause.

"There are two types of ailments [that arise due to] the humours of this life: ailments that arise due to the inherent conditions [of the body] and passing ailments arising from external conditions. The first [arise due to disturbance of] the wind, bile and phlegm, and the second from poisons, weapons and spirits.

(II) WITH RESPECT TO THE TYPE OF PATIENT

"With respect to the patient, there are five divisions: ailments of (A) men, (B) women, (C) children, (D) old people and (E) general illnesses common to all.

(A) MEN

"With respect to men's ailments, there are a decrease and overabundance of semen, swelling of the testicles [as a result of any of the following six causes: disorders of wind, bile, phlegm, fat, urine and the small intestine] and nine [disorders of the] penis:

1. 'brum pa can: formation of small bumps in the urinary tract in the penis
2. mdud pa 'dra ba: formation of knots in the blood vessels in the penis
3. sbubs 'byar ba: retraction of the tip of the penis
4. gra ma can: pain as if there were a thorn in the penis
5-9. disorders due to disturbances of wind, bile, phlegm, blood and any combination of these four.

"[There come to a total of] 17 [types of male disorders].

(B) WOMEN

"With respect to women's ailments, there are five womb [disorders due to disturbances of wind, bile, phlegm, blood and any combination of these four] and nine types of tumours in the womb:

1. chu bur can: tumours that are soft like a bubble and are easy to remove
2. hrem po: hard, tough tumours
3. bem po: hard, resilient tumours that are first small, then grow to a large size
4. rmen skran: a type of tumour found not only in the womb but on the skin and in other organs
5. pho skran: a type of tumour found in the stomach that forms due to a disorder of the blood in the womb
6. skran ro nag po: enlarging of the womb and menstrual disorder due to the growth of extraneous flesh that was not expelled from the womb at childbirth
7. rtsa skran: cancerous inflammation of the blood vessels as a result of a menstrual disorder
8. sa bon gyi skran: a disorder of the ovum which causes it to enlarge cancerously
9. za khu: the formation of a large tumour in the womb such that there appears to be a pregnancy. This is due to a disorder in the fluid that is normally discharged during intercourse.

"Further, there are two disorders of agitation of the organisms in the womb and venereal disease. [It is due to the above organisms that lust arises, and if the lust is not satisfied, mental imbalance may ensue.] Finally, there are 16 types of ailments arising from menstrual disorders.

These are located in the lungs, heart, liver, spleen, gall bladder, kidneys, small intestine, urinary bladder, breasts and large intestine. Ailments that arise due to a disturbance of wind, after menstruation has ceased to occur, in the skull, heart, kidneys, stomach, small intestine and all the hollow organs.

"[These ailments come to a total of] 32.

(C) CHILDREN

"With respect to children's ailments, there are (1) eight subtle, (2) eight coarse and (3) eight very subtle [types of ailments].

1 The eight subtle ailments are of the chest, lungs, liver and navel and include diarrhoea, vomiting, children's contagious diseases and the formation of stones in the kidneys, urinary bladder and genitals.
2 The eight coarse ailments are swelling of the head, disorders of the throat, spleen, gall bladder, stomach and large intestine, ailments due to improper diet and ailments due to improper intercourse of the parents at the time of the child's conception.
3 The eight very subtle ailments are of the eyes, ears, nose, mouth, protrusion of flesh on the skin (rmen bu), the life channel, paralysis due to organisms in the stomach and disorders of the flesh.

(D) OLD PEOPLE

"The ailment of old people is the degeneration of physical strength, which depends upon the five elements of the body.

(E) GENERAL AILMENTS

"With respect to general ailments common to all, there are the classifications of (1) [101 ailments with regard to the three] humours, (2) [101 with regard to] principal ailments, (3) [101 with regard to the] locations [of ailments] and (4) [101 with regard to] general categories [of ailments].

(1) Humour Ailments

"There are three classifications of ailments of the humours: (a) wind, (b) bile and (c) phlegm.

(a) Wind Ailment

"With respect to wind ailments, there are (i) general and (ii) specific disorders.

(i) General

"General disorders are classified with respect to a) type and b) location.

a) Type

There are 20 wind disorders with respect to type (having the following symptoms):

1. *a wa tra*: difficulty in exhaling, wheezing, unclear; memory and awareness, the habit of looking about as if frightened.
2. *da rgan*: protrusion of the breast-bone, together with an upward turning of the neck, or a protrusion of the spine at the first, sixth or seventh vertebra from the top, gritting of the teeth, the appearance of sour, bubbly saliva, inability to speak loudly, frequent yawning and stretching, shooting pain in the ribs.
3. *nang gug*: concaving of the breast-bone and ribs.
4. *'grams pa nyams pa*: intermittent shooting pains in the jawbone, base of the skull and upper back.
5. *lce ldib*: heaviness of the body, inability to speak clearly, difficulty in moving.
6. *phyogs gcig gug pa*: paralysis on one side of the body.
7. *rtsa 'dzin*: falling out of the hair, darkening of the skin on the top of the head and roughness of the skin due to a decrease in the power of the life-supporting wind.
8. *gzhogs phyed skams pa*: thinness, weakness and lack of strength and sensation on one side of the body.
9. *lus kun skams pa*: thinness of the entire body, darkening of the skin, talkativeness.
10. *shing ltar rengs pa*: sudden stiffening of the body such that the patient dies if he is made warm.

11 *dpung pa 'ja' ba:* pain in the shoulders as if they were broken; pain in the armpits.

12 *pi sha rtse:* heat in the palms of the hands, retraction of the ligaments in the fingers making it difficult to stretch them.

13 *sra 'theng:* pain at the base of the back, the testicles and the ligaments on both sides of the scrotum, trembling while walking, walking as if lame or with an upward-jerking motion of the shoulders due to the pain in the above ligaments.

14 *brla rengs:* hardening of the ligaments and pain in the thighs, especially when cold, due to overeating and a surplus of phlegm and fat, difficulty in walking, bodily heaviness.

15 *ce spyang mgo:* swelling of the knees due to a disorder of the wind and blood, causing difficulty in walking.

16 *tsher ma:* pain in the calf bones, shins and ankles as if there were something moving inside these bones, pain in the Achilles' tendon.

17 *gzugs 'kyums:* cramps in the thighs and calves.

18 *kha li:* symptoms like those of no. 12, together with pain in the lower forearms.

19 *skang pa brtse ba:* pain in the soles of the feet while walking, as if treading on sharp stones.

20 *rkang pa tsha ba:* intermittent swelling and heat in the feet while walking.

b) Location

"With respect to location, there are six types of entrances [of wind disorders] and the appearance of the 'flower' [of wind disorders] in the sense organs:

1 wind disturbance in the skin: a feeling as if one's skin is tight, cracked and rough, pain with any kind of bodily contact.

2 wind disturbance in the flesh: aching and swelling of the muscles as if they have been beaten, the appearance of pimples.

3 wind disturbance in the vessels: vessels become as if hollow or they bulge out due to the power of wind entering the blood, complexion turns red or dark, limbs become stiff or else very loose while walking.

4   wind disturbance in the bones: pain in all the bones, thinness, unclear senses, falling of semen, swelling of the joints, stiffening of the neck. Due to the entrance of a wind disturbance into the marrow, one experiences insomnia and a feeling as if one's body were wrapped tightly in a cloth. This feeling is relieved by massage.

5   wind disturbance in the solid organs:

   a   heart: pain in the chest and back, sighing, idle talkativeness.

   b   lungs: swelling of the face, repeated clearing of the throat, with nothing coming up but a little bubbly saliva.

   c   liver: frequent yawning three to four hours after eating, a feeling as if the liver has sunk down a little.

   d   spleen: burping, swelling of the abdomen together with abdominal sounds, pain in the spleen.

   e   kidneys: pain in the bones at the base of the back, difficulty in hearing although nothing is wrong with the ears.

6   wind disturbance in the hollow organs:

   a   upper stomach: burping, swelling of the stomach, great thirst, difficulty in breathing.

   b   middle stomach: shooting pains in and sounds emitted from the large intestine, difficulty in urinating and defecating, pain in the bones directly behind the anus.

   c   gall bladder: poor digestion, yellowing of the whites of the eyes and the nails.

   d   small intestine: dryness of the stool, constipation followed by diarrhoea.

   e   urinary bladder: difficulty in urinating, such that urine is expelled slowly for five minutes or so, swelling of the urinary bladder.

   f   womb: pain during menstruation, with the appearance of only a little blood, or else a strong flow of blood for a longer period than normal.

7   wind disturbance in the sense organs:

a   eyes: reddening of the vessels in the eyes, a feeling as if the eyes are bulging out. These symptoms are worse when one is out in the wind.

b   ears: difficulty in hearing, a roaring sound in the ears, a feeling as if the ears are protruding, shooting pains in the ears.

c   nose: blockage of the nostrils, the appearance of mucus, inability to distinguish odours. As a result of such disorders, one may also experience a loss of sensation in the teeth, swelling of the cheeks, dizziness or a roaring sound in the ears.

(ii) Specific

"There are five kinds of specific [wind disorders] with regard to the life-supporting wind, etc. and 10 [types of disorders involving combinations of wind with] bile and phlegm.

"Symptoms of disorders of the five types of wind are as follows:

1   life-supporting wind: dizziness, talkativeness, difficulty in inhaling, a feeling as if the upper portion of one's body has risen.

2   upward-moving wind: inability to speak clearly and audibly, timidity, physical weakness and poor memory.

3   pervasive wind: much fright, the tendency to speak much at random.

4   fire-accompanying wind: lack of appetite, difficulty in digestion, vomiting.

5   downward-clearing wind: a feeling as if the joints were loose, difficulty in defecating and urinating.

"The 10 combination-disorders involve the first type of wind and the first type of bile, the first type of wind and the first type of phlegm, the second type of wind and the second type of bile, the second type of wind and the second type of phlegm and so on.

"Thus, there are 42 categories of wind disorders.

(b) Bile

"With regard to bile ailments, there are (i) general and (ii) specific disorders.

(i) General

"General disorders are classified with respect to a) type and b) location.

a) Type

There are three types of disorders with respect to type [having the following symptoms]:

1. *thang la lhag pa:* overflowing of bile.
2. *gnas gyur:* movement of bile from the gall bladder to the liver and stomach, where in unusual cases it may form stones.
3. *kha lud and rtsa rgyug:* vomiting of bile due to the formation of stones in the gall bladder; entrance of bile into the blood system, causing yellowing of the eyes and skin.

b) Location

"With regard to location, there are the six entrances and the sense organs:

1. bile disturbance in the skin: yellowing of the skin.
2. bile disturbance in the flesh: decrease in and darkening of the flesh.
3. bile disturbance in the vessels: yellowing of the whites of the eyes.
4. bile disturbance in the bones: thinness and loss of appetite.
5. bile disturbance in the solid organs:

   a. heart: discomfort in the upper region of the trunk, yellowing of the eyes, insomnia, desire for only cool food.
   b. lungs: yellowing of the mucus, coughing especially at noon and midnight.
   c. liver: blue complexion, pain in the liver and heart, a hot, dry feeling in the eyes.
   .d. spleen: the tongue turns blue-green or yellow with streaks of red, bulging of the stomach, pain

in the spleen, swelling of the left leg, pain in all
the joints.

  e   kidneys: heaviness of the body, loss of sensation
       in the legs, pain in the kidneys and hip-bones,
       yellowing of the backs of the ears.

6 bile disturbance in the hollow organs:

  a   stomach: vomiting and evacuation of bile.
  b   large intestine: evacuation of bile.
  c   small intestine: evacuation of bile.
  d   urinary bladder: frequent urination, but little is
       emitted and its colour is dark.
  e   womb: emission of yellow regenerative fluid, the
       formation of tumours in the womb.

7 bile disturbance in the sense organs:

  a   head: headaches during the autumn or as soon
       as one goes out under a hot sun or near a hot
       fire.
  b   eyes: yellowing and a burning feeling in the eyes.
  c   ears: shooting pains and a feeling of heat in the
       ears, the appearance of lymph from the ears.
  d   nose: yellowing of the nose and the skin under
       the eyes, blockage in the upper part of the nose.
  e   tongue: yellowing of the tongue, a bitter taste in
       the mouth.

(ii) Specific

"There are five kinds of specific [bile disorders] with regard to the
digestive bile, etc. and 10 [types of disorders involving combinations of bile with] wind and phlegm.

"Symptoms of disorders of the five types of bile are as follows:

1 digestive bile: with the decrease of the power of the
   digestive bile, the fire-accompanying wind is unable
   to separate the chyle from the inferior sediment, and
   this causes the stomach to bulge and the stool to become dry.
2 colour-transforming bile: itching and yellowing of the
   skin.
3 accomplishing bile: unclear memory and awareness,
   need of much sleep.

    4 visually-operating bile: one is unable to gaze at the sun and sees white objects as yellow.

    5 complexion-clearing bile: the skin turns rough and dark blue, the hair of the head and the eyebrows fall out, the body loses strength and the fingernails turn dark.

"The 10 combination-disorders involve the five types of bile paired off with the five types of phlegm.

Thus, there are 26 categories of bile disorders.

(c) Phlegm

"There are two types of phlegm disorders: (i) simple and (ii) complex.

    Simple phlegm disorders involve primarily a disturbance of phlegm alone, whereas complex disorders begin as a simple disorder but lead to another more serious ailment of a different nature.

    (i) Simple Disorder

'With regard to simple disorders, there are a) general and b) specific illnesses.

    a) General

'General illnesses are classified with respect to i) type and ii) location.

      i) Type

There are six categories in terms of type.

    1 *lhen:* a disorder in the upper region of the stomach due to an over-accumulation of mucus there. It results in loss of appetite, a feeling as if there were something firm and round in the upper region of the stomach, and poor digestion. The symptoms are felt immediately after eating.

    2 *lcags dregs:* a disorder that arises due to an over-accumulation of mucus in the stomach. It results in stomach ulcers, frequent belching, a very full feeling in the stomach, loss of weight, lassitude and occasional vomiting of sour fluid.

    3 *me nyams:* a disorder involving complete inability to digest food, bulging and emission of sound from the

stomach, frequent belching of bad-smelling air four to five hours after eating, diarrhoea soon after eating if the downward-clearing wind is strong, loss of weight and much accumulation of water in the stomach resulting in protrusion of the stomach as well as the formation of stomach tumours.

4. *mgul 'gags:* blockage of the throat due to an accumulation of phlegm in the lungs. This results in difficulty in breathing, speaking and swallowing, loss of weight and strength, and reduction of the size of the stomach. This is particularly difficult to cure.

5. *grum bu:* a disorder in the stomach and liver due to poor digestion. It results in an inability to distinguish tastes, alternating vomiting and diarrhoea, pain in the lower arms and legs and lower forehead, frequent vomiting of fluid, and stiffening of the joints such that movement of the limbs is painful.

6. *'jum skem:* a disorder that arises due to an over-accumulation of organisms related to phlegm. Because these organisms consume most of the nourishment in one's food, one experiences an insatiable appetite and under-nourishment, loss of weight and strength, bulging of the stomach, trembling of the calves if one remains standing, and lassitude.

ii) Location

"The categories in terms of location are the six entrances and the sense organs:

1. phlegm disturbance in the skin: low bodily heat, paleness and flakiness of the skin, and general itching.

2. phlegm disturbance in the flesh: low bodily heat, dark facial complexion, dark splotches on the skin, much sleep, heaviness of the body, lassitude and small tumours on the skin.

3. phlegm disturbances in the vessels: constant coldness of the body, firmness of the flesh as if the muscles were tensed, and heaviness of the body.

4. phlegm disturbance in the bones: a cold feeling in the bones, pain and slight swelling in the joints causing pain when the limbs are extended and retracted.

5. phlegm disturbance in the solid organs:

   a. heart: mental dullness, loss of appetite, a full feeling in the chest and heaviness of body and mind.
   b. lungs: a feeling of fullness in the chest, dizziness and the coughing up of dark blue phlegm.
   c. liver: pain in the liver immediately after eating and the emission of nutriment [in the form of bluish liquid] from the mouth due to the inability of the liver to receive it.
   d. spleen: heavy breathing, bulging of the abdomen, weakness, lassitude and the passing of stools having the same colour as that of the food eaten.
   e. kidneys: pain in the hips, very frequent urination and difficulty in hearing.

6. phlegm disturbance in the hollow organs:

   a. stomach: lack of appetite, heaviness of the body and a feeling of heat in the breast-bone.

   b. large intestine: bulging and emission of sound from the abdomen and discomfort immediately after eating.

   c. small intestine: much mucus in the stool and heaviness of the body.

   d. gall bladder: yellowing of the whites of the eyes, poor digestion, heaviness of the body, lassitude, much sleep and mental dullness.

   e. urinary bladder: emission of sperm as when one has diabetes.

   f. reproductive organs: a woman passes an abundance of menstrual blood, and a man feels a hot pain in the tip of the penis while urinating and sperm is emitted.

7 phlegm disturbance in the sense organs:

   a. head: heaviness of the head, much sleep and lack of appetite.
   b. eyes: slight swelling of the skin under the eyes and the falling of tears.

c. ears: coldness and a feeling of heaviness of the ears and difficulty in hearing.
d. nose: blockage of the nostrils and heaviness of the upper cheeks.
e. tongue: inability to distinguish tastes and a thick feeling in the tongue resulting in difficulty in speaking.

a) Specific

"There are five kinds of specific [phlegm disorders] with regard to the supportive phlegm, etc., and 10 [types of disorders involving combinations of phlegm with] wind and bile.

"Symptoms of disorders of the five types of phlegm are as follows:

1 supportive phlegm: lack of appetite, a full feeling in the chest, shooting pains in the upper trunk, a feeling of heat in the breast-bone and frequent vomiting of sour fluid.
2 mixing phlegm: poor digestion, vomiting of any kind of food as soon as it is taken, frequent belching, and tightness of the abdomen.
3 experiencing phlegm: inability to distinguish tastes, lack of thirst, a cold feeling in the tongue, the upper lip turns up and the lower turns down, and roughness of the voice.
4 satisfying phlegm: a feeling of heaviness on one side of the head, visual distortion, blockage of the ears, frequent sneezing, emission of fluid from the nose, a heavy feeling in the top of the head and frequent influenza.
5 connecting phlegm: difficulty in extending and retracting the limbs, thickness of the joints, a loose feeling and pain in the shoulders and hip joints, and swelling of all the joints.

"The 10 combination-disorders involve the five types of phlegm paired off with the five types of wind and five types of bile.

(ii) Complex

"With regard to complex [phlegm disorders, there are the following types]:

1 *ser po:* phlegm disorders combined with a strong element of bile.

2 *smug po:* phlegm disorders combined with a strong element of blood.

3 *smug po byer ba:* a disorder having two varieties, external and internal. The former pervades the flesh, skin, fat and vessels, and the latter affects the heart, lungs, spleen and kidneys. They are associated with both hot and cold disorders and bear symptoms like those of a wind disorder. A hot or cold environment and diet worsen the disorder.

4 *smug po rgyas pa:* a disorder similar to a simple phlegm disorder and involving coughing, pain in the heart, strained breathing, vibration of the head hair, loss of colour in the lips and nails, yellowing of the upper cheeks, strong thirst and the desire to consume cool food and drink.

5 *smug po rdol ba:* a disorder involving a hot feeling in the chest and much vomiting of blood and a dark fluid.

6 *smug po 'gyings pa:* a disorder involving pain in the diaphragm, belching, a feeling as if one's breath is sweet, inability to distinguish tastes, much perspiration, frequent poor digestion, a tight feeling in the stomach, dryness of the stool and the formation of tumours. The symptoms are relieved somewhat by vomiting.

"Thus, there are 33 categories of phlegm disorders, making a total of 101 categories of disorders of the humours.

(2) Principal Ailments

"Principal ailments have the categories of (a) simple and (b) complex.

(a) Simple

"Simple disorders bear the symptoms of [a disturbance of only] one of the humours. These involve (1) an increase, (2) strong increase, (3) violent increase, (4) decrease, (5) strong decrease and (6) violent decrease [of any of the three humours, thus making a total of 18 categories].

(b) Complex

"Complex disorders involve (i) dual and (ii) triple combinations of the humours and (iii) delicate ailments.

(i) Dual Combination

"Dual combinations. There are three categories of parallel disorders [for both increase and decrease of the humours] and six categories of combinations in which one [of the humours] strongly [increases or decreases] and another [increases or decreases] yet more strongly.

These include the following: Similar increases or decreases of both (1, 2) wind and bile, (3, 4) phlegm and bile, (5, 6) phlegm and wind. Strong increase or decrease of the former humour combined with a yet stronger increase or decrease of the latter: (7, 8) wind and bile, (9, 10) bile and phlegm, (11, 12) phlegm and wind, (13, 14) bile and wind, (15, 16) phlegm and bile, and (17, 18) wind and phlegm.

(ii) Triple Combination

"Triple combinations. Among these are first included similar [(1)increases and (2) decreases of all three humours]. There are six combinations [with regard to both increase and decrease of the humours] involving a strong [increase or decrease of the humour listed first], a medium [increase or decrease of the second] and a minor [increase or decrease of the third: (3, 4) wind, bile and phlegm, (5, 6) bile, phlegm and wind, (7, 8) phlegm, wind and bile, (9, 10) wind, phlegm and bile, (11, 12) bile, wind and phlegm, (13, 14) phlegm, bile and wind]. There are six combinations with regard to [an increase as well as] a decrease [of the humours] involving two [sets of humours] in which [the change in the latter] one is stronger [and of the same kind as the former: (15, 16) wind, phlegm and bile, (17, 18) bile, phlegm and wind, (19, 20) phlegm, bile and wind, (21, 22) bile and wind, phlegm, (23, 24) phlegm and bile, wind, (25, 26) phlegm and wind, bile]. There are six combinations involving both decrease and increase [of the humours] in the following manner: the humour listed first weakens, the second increases and the third decreases: (27) wind, bile and phlegm, (28) bile, phlegm and wind, (29) phlegm, wind and bile, (30) phlegm, bile and wind, (31) bile, phlegm and wind, (32) wind, phlegm and bile. Finally, there are six [combinations] in which the first [set of humours listed] decreases and the second increases: [(33) wind; bile and phlegm, (34) bile; phlegm and wind, (35) phlegm; wind and bile, (36) wind and bile; phlegm, (37) phlegm and bile; wind and (38) phlegm and wind; bile]. Thus there are 74 divisions with regard to increases and decreases [of the humours].

(iii) Delicate Combinations

"There are also three divisions of delicate ailments involving the arising of one disorder on top of another [i.e. before the former has been healed]: a) entrance [of one or two humours in the location of another], b) disturbance [of one or two humours before a disorder of another has been healed] and c) mixture [of the humours].

a) Entrance

"The entrance of [the latter] humour(s) into the location of the former: [(1) wind; bile, (2) wind; phlegm, (3) wind; bile and phlegm, (4) bile; wind, (5) bile; phlegm, (6) bile; wind and phlegm, (7) phlegm; wind, (8) phlegm; bile and (9) phlegm; wind and bile].

b) Disturbance

"A disturbance of [the latter] humour(s) before [the disorder of] the first has been healed: [(10) wind; bile, (11) wind; phlegm, (12) wind; bile and phlegm, (13) bile; wind, (14) bile; phlegm, (15) bile; wind and phlegm, (16) phlegm; wind, (17) phlegm; bile and (18) phlegm; bile and wind].

c) Mixture

"A mixture of two types of humours: [(19) a mixture of phlegm and bile in the location of the wind, (20) a mixture of phlegm and wind in the location of the bile after the displacement of the bile by the wind, (21) a mixture of bile and wind in the location of the phlegm after the displacement of the phlegm by the wind, (22) a mixture of phlegm and wind in the location of the bile, (23) a mixture of phlegm and bile in the location of the wind after the wind has been displaced by the bile, (24) a mixture of bile and wind in the location of the phlegm after the phlegm has been displaced by the bile, (25) a mixture of wind and bile in the location of the phlegm, (26) a mixture of phlegm and bile in the location of the wind after the wind has been displaced by the phlegm, and (27) a mixture of phlegm and wind in the location of the bile after the bile has been displaced by the phlegm]. Thus, there are three sets of nine.

"These total 101 categories of principal disorders.

(3) *Location of Ailments*

"With regard to location, there are the two divisions of body and mind. There are two [disorders] that are located in the mind—insanity and loss of memory. [Disorders that are] located in the body [are found] in the (a) upper, (b) inner (c) lower and (d) outer [areas of the body]. There is also a fifth category including ailments that are found in all [areas of the body], external and internal.

(a) Upper

"[Disorders] located in the upper region of the body in the sense organs and the head [are found specifically in the following areas]: (1) head, (2) eyes, (3) ears, (4) nose, (5) lips, (6) teeth, (7) tongue, (8) palate and (9) goitre, throat and the region from the base of the throat to the top of the head. [Disorders of] the throat include (10) ailments [such as tonsillitis], (11) blockage [due to the formation of tumours in the throat], (12) throat blockage [due to a constriction of the throat] and (13) speech impediments. [Disorders that are] located generally in the region from base of the throat to the top of the head include: (14) abnormal thirst, (15) hiccoughs, (16) asthma [of five varieties], (17) difficulty in swallowing such that food sticks in the chest region and (18) the common cold [of which there are five varieties]. These come to a total of 18.

(b) Inner

"[Disorders] located in the solid and hollow organs [are found in the following areas]: (1) heart [four types of ailments], (2) lungs [eight types of ailments], (3) liver [four types of ailments], (4) spleen [two types of ailments], (5) kidneys [five types of ailments], (6) stomach [six types of ailments], (7) gall bladder [two types of ailments], (8) small intestine [three types of ailments], (9) large intestine [two types of ailments], (10) urinary bladder [three types of ailments], (11) vesicle of regenerative fluid [two types of ailments]. [Disorders] located generally in the solid and hollow organs include: (12) poor digestion [of three varieties, all of which affect the other organs besides the stomach], (13) ailments [of three varieties] due to organisms in the abdomen (glang thabs), (14) tumours [of two varieties], (15) cancerous sores (sur ya), (16) diarrhoea relating to a heat disorder and (17) dysentery [of three varieties]. [Disorder located generally in the hollow organs include: (18) diarrhoea [of two varieties] and (19) vomiting [of two varieties]. These come to a total of 19 types of disorders.

(c) Lower

"Disorders in the lower region of the body include:
1. haemorrhoids [of five types]
2. *mtshan bar rdol ba:* an ailment [of two varieties] involving the appearance of a hole between the anus and the genitals
3. constipation [of two types]
4. urine blockage [of two types]
5. *grin snyi:* a disorder [having two varieties] such that the urine is expelled only at a slow rate.

(d) Outer

"[Disorders] located in the outer region of the body are [found in] the skin, flesh, vessels and bones. Skin ailments include:
1. *sha bkra:* blotchiness of the skin
2. *bas ldags:* a disorder involving external sores and flaking of the skin
3. *g yan pa:* a disorder involving a prickling sensation in the skin and flaking of the skin when scratched
4. *glang shu:* a disorder involving sores all over the skin
5. *za kong:* a disorder involving itching all over the body. There are two varieties of all the above skin disorders.
6. *shu ba:* a disorder [having three varieties] involving recurring sores on the skin
7. *reg pa'i dug:* venereal disorders [of three varieties]
8. *mdzer pa:* a contagious disorder [having 18 varieties] involving sores all over the skin, especially around the eyes, which results in the loss of the eyebrows
9. *ngo khebs:* a disorder [of two varieties] involving a darkening of the skin around the eyes
10. other ailments that spread in the skin.

"Ailments of the flesh include:
11. goitre [of eight types]
12. *rmen bu:* small bumps on the skin [of two varieties]
13. other ailments that spread in the flesh.

"Ailments of the vessels include [disorders of the]:
14. lymphatic vessels [of four kinds]
15. blood vessels [of two kinds]

16. other disorders that move in the vessels.

"Bone ailments include:

17. *dreg:* a disorder [having four varieties] involving pain in the joints in the bottom of the feet
18. *rkang bam:* a disorder [having three varieties] of the bones from the hips down to the feet
19. other disorders that cling to the bones
20. *grum bu:* a disorder [having five varieties] located in all the bones and flesh and involving deformity of the limbs.

"These come to a total of 20.

(e) External and Internal

"The category of ailments found in all the external and internal [areas of the body] includes:

1. *mkhris pa:* bile disorders
2. *smug po:* phlegm disorders combined with a strong element of blood [one form of tuberculosis]
3. *dmu:* protrusion of the stomach due to an accumulation of water there. This and other ailments involving an accumulation of water occur as a result of poor digestive heat.
4. *'or:* a disorder involving swelling of the side of the body facing down while sleeping
5. *skya rbab:* a disorder that precedes *'or.* Its symptoms are slight swelling of the legs just above the ankles, swelling of the eyes and loss of colour in the cheeks.
6. *gcong:* the accumulation in the liver and lungs of a mixture of nutriment with blood and bile. This occurs due to poor digestion and is very difficult to heal because any treatment given leads to another disorder.
7. *tsha ba ma smin:* heat disorders involving shivering and pain in all the joints
8. *tsha ba rgyas pa:* heat disorders involving such a high temperature that the body feels as if it is on fire
9. *tsha ba stongs pa:* heat disorders with which the temperature appears externally to be higher than it actually is, due to agitation by the winds

10 *tsha ba gab pa:* heat disorders that are hidden in the heart [easily mistaken for a disorder of the life-supporting wind], kidneys [easily mistaken for a cold disorder] or stomach [easily mistaken for a digestive disorder]

11 *tsha ba rnyings pa:* chronic heat ailments that cling to the vessels and bones

12 *tsha ba rnyongs ba:* heat disorders that are mixed with various stages of chyle [as the chyle passes through the digestive cycle]

13 *'grams tshad:* a mixture of lymph and blood due to violent physical exertion or an accident while suffering from a heat disorder. This especially affects the solid organs or the skin and flesh such that the latter feel as if they are being beaten.

14 *'khrugs tshad:* a disturbance of all three humours due to an increase in the power of the blood, resulting in a feeling of heat throughout the body

15 *rims tshad:* contagious heat ailments arising due to an increase in the power of the digestive bile. These are more pravalent nowadays due to the mass production of nuclear devices and motor-driven vehicles and to the low standard of morality in the world.

16 *'brum bu:* the six types of poxes

17 *lhog pa:* a disorder involving swelling of the limbs, the emission of pus, and high temperature

18 poisoning from artificial poison

19 poisoning from substances carried in the air [e.g. from a nuclear explosion]

20 poisoning from spirits, resulting in shooting pains

21 poisoning from vapours [e.g. from boiling mercury]

22 meat poisoning

23 poisoning from unwholesome food combinations

24 poisoning from an extremely toxic plant bearing the name of *btsan dug*

25 rabies

26 poisoning from scorpions, spiders, etc.

27 snake poisoning

28 disorders inflicted by a type of spirit (*'byung po*)

29 disorders caused by planetary influence

30 leprosy

31 *'bras:* chronic sores on the skin which eventually result in the softening of the bone beneath

32 me dbal: the appearance of red sores all over the body
    due to impure blood in the liver
33 disorders involving itching all over the body due to
    organisms in the system
34 head sores
35 sores on the trunk from the waist up to the neck
36 sores on the limbs
37 neck sores.

"These come to a total of 37 and a grand total of 101 [categories of ailments] with regard to location.

(4) General Catagories of Ailments

"With regard to general categories, there are the divisions of (a) internal ailments from the waist up to the neck, (b) sores, (c) heat disorders and (d) miscellaneous disorders.

(a) Internal Ailments

"Internal trunk disorders include poor digestion and the chronic ailments (gcong nad) that result therefrom. Poor digestion is classified with regard to its nature, category [of foods that cannot be digested], accompanying disorder and stage. The resulting chronic ailments are classified into (i) new and (ii) old.

(i) New

"New chronic disorders are divided into the phlegm disorders a) skya bo and b) smug po, c) bile disorders and d) chronic ailments due to poisoning.

a) skya bo

"The category of phlegm disorders called skya bo includes: (1) lhen, (2) lcags dreg, (3) me nyams, (4) mgul 'gags, (5) grum bu dkar po, and (6) 'ju skem.

b) smugpo

"The category of phlegm disorders called smug po includes:

1-3 byer ba, rgyas pa, rdol ba
  4 ral: a disorder involving the bursting of the vessels in
     the liver and much vomiting of blood
  5 gyings pa
  6 'gril: congestion of blood in the liver or stomach

7 *gab:* a form of tuberculosis that is hidden in the blood, making it difficult to recognize unless it manifests itself in the liver or stomach

8 *'thab:* a disorder involving a mixture of phlegm and heat

9 *'or lhung:* thinness and bodily weakness due to a serious phlegm disorder

10 *grang ba lhing chad:* complete exhaustion of the power of phlegm

c) Bile Disorders

"Bile disorders include: (1) *kha lud,* (2) *rtsa rguyg* and (3) *gnas gyur.*

d) Chronic Ailments

"Chronic ailments due to poisoning include disorders due to poisons prepared with hot and cold substances.

(ii) Old

"Old chronic ailments are divided into a) tumours *(skran),* b) *dmu,* c) *'or,* d) *skya rbab* and e) *gcong chen zad byed.*

a) Tumours

"The eight types of tumours include:

1 tumours in the vessels
2 tumours in the gall bladder
3 tumours in the upper region of the stomach
4 stone-like tumours
5 rubbery tumours occurring primarily in the large intestine and heart due to wind disorders
6 tumours that form from the accumulation of dead organisms in the body
7 tumours in the large intestine that form due to an obstruction of excrement
8 tumours that form in the canal between the kidneys and urinary bladder due to an obstruction in the flow of urine.

b) dmu

"*dmu* disorders include:

1 *dmu chu byer:* swelling of the entire body with water, due to poor digestion

2 *zags:* falling of water from the lungs down to the liver and kidneys

3 *'khyims chu:* bulging of the hollow organs due to an accumulation of water

4 *rdol chu:* cracking of the skin followed by the emission of lymph

c) 'or

'or disorders include those related to heat and cold ailments.

d) skya rbab

skya rbab disorders include those related to disorders of the lungs, heart, liver, spleen and lymph.

e) gcong chen zad byed

gcong chen zad byed disorders [problematic ailments involving a decrease in the power of the bodily constituents and an increase in the power of the lymph and the accompanying disorder] are of four types [those related with a disturbance of] wind, bile, phlegm or a delicate ailment.

(b) Sores

"Sores include (i) those arising from internal disorders and (ii) those inflicted externally.

(i) Internal Disorder

"Sores arising due to internal disorders include:

1 *'bras:* chronic sores on the skin which eventually result in the softening of the bone beneath

2 *rmen bu:* protrusions of flesh on the skin that become cancerous if not treated

3 *sur ya:* sores in the solid and hollow organs that become cancerous if not treated. These may arise due to improper diet or as a result of a contagious disease.

4 *me dbal:* the appearance of red sores all over the body due to impure blood in the liver

5 haemorrhoids

6 *rkang bam:* a disorder of the bones from the hips down to the feet

7 *mtshan bar drol ba:* an ailment involving the appearance of a hole between the anus and the genitals.

(ii) External

"Externally inflicted sores are classified in terms of location and category. The locations include the head, neck, trunk and limbs. The categories of sores include: (1) peeling [of the skin], (2) cutting [of the skin], (3) complete severing [of muscles], (4) partial severing [of muscles], (5) loss [of limbs, etc.], (6) complete piercing [of any part of the body], (7) splitting [of flesh] and (8) cracking [of the bones].

"These come to a total of 15 categories.

(c) Heat Disorders

"Heat disorders include: (1) *tsha ba ma smin*, (2)   *tsha ba rgyas pa*, (3) *tsha ba stongs pa*, (4) *tsha ba gab pa*, (5) *tsha ba rnyings pa* and (6) *tsha ba rnyongs pa* as well as the four categories of *'grams tshad*, *'khrugs tshad*, contagious heat disorders and heat disorders due to poisoning. The ailment *'grams tshad* is of two kinds—(7) outer [affecting the skin and flesh] and (8) inner [affecting the solid organs]. There are three types of *'khrugs tshad:*

9. *rgyas 'khrugs*: a heat ailment involving a disturbance of all three humours due to strong physical exertion while suffering from a disturbance of blood and bile
10. *stong 'khrugs*: a disturbance of all three humours with a strong wind element due to improper behaviour while an old heat ailment is gradually healing
11. *'jam 'khrugs:* a mild heat disorder combined with a strong element of phlegm.

"The five types of contagious heat disorders include:

12. *bal nad*: an ailment similar to dysentery
13. *rgyu gzer:* a type of dysentery that becomes critical if not treated quickly
14. poxes
15. *gag lhog:* a disorder involving swelling of the throat and the appearance of sores on the throat from which pus emerges
16. the common cold.

"The three types of poisoning are those resulting from: (17) manufactured poisons, (18) substances that turn into poison [e.g. meat when left in a warm, moist place] and (19) natural poisons.

(d) Miscellaneous Disorders

"Miscellaneous disorders include: (1) blockage of the throat, (2) hiccoughs, (3) blockage of food in the area of the chest, (4) abnormal thirst, (5) asthma, (6) glang thabs [ailments due to organisms in the abdomen], (7) disorders involving itching due to organisms in the body, (8) diarrhoea, (9) vomiting, (10) constipation, (11) blockage of the flow of urine, (12) a urine disorder involving only a slow emission of urine, (13) diarrhoea related to a heat disorder (14) dreg (a disrder involving protrusions of flesh on the soles of the feet), (15) grum bu (a crippling disorder involving pain in all the joints), (16) lymph disorders, (17) disorders of the lymphatic vessels, (18) skin disorders and (19) minor ailments.

'Thus there are 101 divisions [of ailments in terms] of general categories and 404 disorders falling into the four divisions of humours, principal ailments, locations and general categories. Among these there are disorders that result in death even if treated, ailments inflicted by spirits that can be cured through religious practice [followed by proper medication], ailments that result in death if not treated but can be healed with treatment and, finally, minor ailments that heal naturally without medication. If these four [types] are taken into account for each of the 404 [categories of ailments], there comes a total of 1,616 [divisions].

> There are yet further ways of classification giving totals of 1,263,600 and 8,234,400 divisions. These are discussed in the Oral Tradition Tantra (Man ngag gi rgyud) and its commentary Man ngag lhan thabs.

(C) Characteristics of Illness

"There are countless divisions with respect to the characteristics [of illness]. There are 25 humours and objects harmed [i.e. the bodily constituents and impurities] and many types of single, dual and triple disorders. Thus there are no enumeration nor names given to them all. Nevertheless, there are no more than three humours, and there are no locations of disorders other than the 10 objects that can be harmed. For example, wherever a bird may fly, there is no place for it to go but in the sky. Since phlegm and wind are cold and blood and bile are hot, despite the many divisions [of ailments], they are all included in hot and cold disorders.

"With individual subjects [i.e. disorders] there are the cause, early stage, evident stage and fully manifest stage. The cause is the condition that produced [the illness]. The early stage occurs while the symptoms are not yet clear. The evident stage occurs when they become clear, and the fully manifesting stage occurs when [the disorder has] fully ripened [and all the symptoms are evident in their] proper locations.

"With regard to these [disorders], the enumeration, identified [ailments], [the divisions of] principal ailments and the force [of the illness are all taken into account by the physician]. The enumeration is of the [404] divisions of particular types of disorders. The identified [ailments] are those which are unmixed [i.e. simple disorders], but the principal ailments include both simple and complex disorders. These include initial disorders and delicate ailments. The force of an illness is influenced by the environment, time, nature [of individual people] and age groups as well as the type [of individuals in terms] of the humours, and diet and behaviour."

Everyone living on this planet has taken birth in dependence upon the five elements. We rely upon them for the necessities of life and, likewise, all medicines are composed of the five elements.

CHAPTER THIRTEEN

Continual Daily Behaviour

Then Sage Yilé Kyé asked: "O great sage, Rigpé Yeshé, how may we learn about the principle of behaviour? We request the physician, the Sovereign Healer, to explain." The teacher replied: "O great sage, listen! The teaching on the principle of behaviour that acts as a healing factor involves: (I) continual behaviour, (II) seasonal behaviour and (III) occasional behaviour.

(I) "The activity of continual daily behaviour is [of two types], (A) worldly [activities that are conducted for the benefits] of this life only and (B) sacred activities.

(A) "The behaviour [directed towards] this life alone [is explained as follows]: for the sake of continual happiness and long life, there are the supreme medicines, precious stones and minerals and the wearing of tantric amulets.

> The supreme medicines primarily include the 'precious pills' (rin chen ril bu) containing mercury, but also include the medicines a ru ra rnam par rgyal ba, tsha sbyor, grang sbyor and dbang po ril bu as well as shu dag, yungs kar and gu gul, which are worn on the left shoulder as a protection against spirits. The precious stones and minerals include diamond, lapis-lazuli, ruby, sapphire, emerald, gold and silver, etc. Tantric amulets are worn around the neck and may contain a variety of objects that have been blessed with mantras.

"Always avoid the two conditions leading to illness [i.e. unwholesome diet and behaviour] by means of mindfulness. Avoid harmful actions of the body, speech and mind and devote yourselves to what is right. Neither torment your senses of taste and so forth, nor over-indulge in sensual pleasures. Avoid sailing in uncertain [waters], riding untamed animals, travelling in areas of killing [e.g. those inhabited by bandits], entering large bodies of water or places on fire, and climbing on canyon walls and on treetops during the monsoon and winter [when the branches are either slippery or brittle]. When staying in one place, examine it and, when moving, examine your path. [It is better not to travel] by night, [but if it is necessary for some important reason, carry a stick and [go] with a companion.

"Because it is rough [on the internal winds] if one does not sleep at night, sleep in whatever [position] is comfortable. If one does not sleep at night [e.g. due to having much work] refrain from eating the following morning and sleep for half [the normal duration of a night's sleep]. Due to the roughness [in terms of the internal winds] and short nights in early summer, it is beneficial to sleep [for a short time] in the afternoon and [eat] heavy, oily [foods] if one has been intoxicated, is very weak, is exhausted due to sorrow or strenuous effort, if one has been speaking a great deal, if one is old or if one has been frightened. However, if such is not the case, sleeping during the day leads to an increase of phlegm, bagginess [of the skin], mental dullness, headaches, lassitude and tendency to contagious diseases. If one is sleeping too much, [take medicine to induce] vomiting, fast, and enjoy the company of women. For insomnia drink milk, curd, alcohol and meat broth. Anoint the head [and body with sesamum oil] and pour [a drop of] oil into [each of] the ears.

"Refrain from sexual intercourse with non-humans, another's spouse, a person who is unpleasing [to oneself], a pregnant [woman or one who is] weak, ill or having her menstrual period [for this may cause illness for both the man and woman]. [Because] the sperm is strong during the winter, there is no restriction [as to the frequency of sexual intercourse, but during the] autumn, [intercourse should be no more often than once] every two days and during early summer and monsoon [no more than once] in a fortnight. Otherwise, [more frequent] intercourse with women leads to a dulling of the senses, dizziness and premature death.

"Continual application [of oil on the body and proper massage] conquers aging, tiredness and wind ailments. [Occasionally rubbing oil] on the head, feet and ears leads to physical lightness, loss of fat, [physical] well-being and an increase of bodily heat. The ability to have sexual intercourse and perform work comes from giving effort to [the above] proper behaviour. [However], by over-indulging [in sexual intercourse, sleeping, etc.] or engaging in them incorrectly, [the body] becomes unfit. Old people, children and those suffering from wind or bile [disorders or both, should especially] avoid such [unwholesome behaviour].

"People prone to phlegm ailments should do physical exercise, and strong people and those who eat oily [rich] food should do so in the winter and spring. [Afterwards], one should [rub oil on the body, and then when perspiration has appeared], apply [lentil flour all over the skin]. [Finally], dry [the body by rubbing it with a towel]. This rids [the body of excessive] phlegm, aids the digestion of fat, [gives] a clear complexion and is the best [means] for strengthening the limbs [and making them supple].

"[Frequent] bathing gives greater virility, bodily heat, strength, [long] life and [lively] complexion and dispels itching due to perspiration, lassitude, thirst and overheating of the body. Washing the head with warm water causes a loss of hair and visual strength. Those suffering from diarrhoea due to a heat disorder, bloating of the abdomen [e.g. due to poor digestion], a common cold, poor digestion or nose or eye ailments should avoid [bathing] immediately after eating.

"The eyes, being of the nature of fire element, cause a decline of phlegm, which results in the falling of tears. For this one should apply the eye medicine skyer khanda [to the eyes] continuously once every seven days [especially in the winter]. Against the enemies of the five sudden illnesses call on the 'friends'.

> The five illnesses are (1) large swellings on the side of the head (gag pa), (2) appendicitis (pho log), (3) twisting of the lower limbs (nyva log), (4) a type of large swelling anywhere on the body [lhog pa] and (5) the emission of blood from the nose (sna khrag). If any of these ailments appears, one should immediately see a skilled physician. The "friends" refer to the supreme medicines, precious stones and minerals and tantric amulents mentioned above.

"Apply yourself to following not [only] one, but all [of the above advice]. Thus one [casts] suffering far away by the continual close application of mindfulness night and day, while abiding or travelling.

"Living in accordance with the religions of the world is the foundation of all virtues. [Listen] carefully to whatever is said and give a meaningful reply. Even if [others] tell [you to perform some] bad action, turn away from it, and even if [they] obstruct a good action, follow it through. Before [acting], examine [the situation], then act skilfully and with conviction. Do not accept a lot of talk as being true until you have examined it well. Think about the many things [you say], then speak, emphasising the essential points [you wish to express].

"Do not listen to the talk of women nor disclose your secrets [to them]. To those who love [you] or look [to you with hope] speak straightforwardly without deceit. [Let your actions of the body, speech and mind] be controlled and disciplined, and when in the company of others, enjoy yourself. Do not be obstinate with [your] enemies, rather put the conflict in the back [of your mind and gradually, calmly] solve [the problem] with [skilful] means. Care for your friends and relatives with affection and long remember the previous kindness [of others towards yourself]. Respectfully serve [your] teachers and guru, father and uncles. Let [your] thoughts be in harmony with [your] countrymen, friends and those with whom you must live. Be thrifty in your farming [and your wealth in general], but in time of need, give freely. [In any kind of activity if you see] a mistake [on your part, acknowledge your failure, and [if you] have success, be satisfied. If you are learned, subdue your pride, and if you are wealthy, be content. Do not look down upon the lowly and avoid jealousy towards those above you. Do not form close relationships with bad people, and do not become enemies with priests or sorcerers. Do not crave the possessions of others, and give up harmful retaliation and making oaths. [In any kind of activity] walk firmly in order to avoid [later] regret, and do not entrust power to bad people. Establish the foundation of sincere courage, forbearance and broadmindedness, and gladly take on various works at their proper times. Even if such a person is born alone [i.e. as a single child in a family in the next life], he will not lose his power to others. Even if born with the body of a servant [i.e. born in a lowly household], he will become the master of many.

(B) "Sacred religious behaviour [is explained as follows]: because all creatures seek happiness, they engage in all [sorts of] activities. But without a religious approach to life, happiness itself is a cause of discontent. Therefore, apply yourself to a religious way of life. Sincerely devote yourself to a [spiritual] friend and assiduously avoid others [i.e. those who lead others away from truth]. With your body, speech and mind avoid the 10 harmful actions of (1) killing, (2) stealing, (3) sexual misconduct, (4) lying, (5) idle gossip, (6) abusive speech, (7) slanderous speech, (8) covetousness, (9) malice and (10) misguided views. As much as you are able, be of service to those who are filled with misery, the ill, the poor and those in pain. Always look upon all [creatures] such as insects as being similar to yourself [in that we all seek happiness and wish to avoid pain]. Gently smile [upon others] without deceit and speak truthfully. Primarily be of service [to others], even your enemies who strive to harm you. By means of loving kindness, cultivate the two fully awakened states of mind.

The first of these is the heartfelt desire to attain full enlightenment in order to be of greatest service to others. A fully enlightened being is most capable of leading others away from suffering and discontent because he has attained the fulfilment of compassion, wisdom and power. The second state of mind referred to here is that which actively sets about to attain this perfection by following the way of life taught by fully enlightened beings of the past, such as Buddha Shakyamuni.

"Subdue [the actions of your] body, speech and mind and have a generous attitude free of attachment. Also, think of the welfare of others as being similar to your own [i.e. not attaching greater value to the welfare of yourself over that of another]. These are the ideals of religious behaviour."

CHAPTER FOURTEEN

Seasonal Behaviour

Then Sage Rigpé Yeshé spoke thus: "O great sage, listen! Secondly, [the explanation of] seasonal behaviour [is as follows]:

(II) "[The six seasons of the year are] (1) early winter, (2) late winter, (3) spring, (4) early summer, (5) late summer, or monsoon, and (6) autumn. Each is accorded two months."

> In terms of the solar calendar, early winter begins roughly in mid-October and lasts until mid-December. The other five seasons follow accordingly.

"[Measurements of time are as follows] : (1) an instant (skad cig), (2) a moment (thang cig), (3) an hour (yud tsam), (4) a day and night, (5) a month, (6) a season and (7) a year.

> One instant lasts 120 times the duration of a subtle thought. There are 60 instants per moment, 30 moments per hour, 30 hours per day and night, 30 days and nights per month, two months per season and six seasons per year.

"The sun turns about [i.e. the period of daylight begins to increase and decrease] in mid-summer and mid-winter 11 days [after the lunar date of the solstices of the immediately preceding year]. [After turning about], it is said to move south [after the summer solstice] and north [after the winter solstice for the duration of] three [seasons]. When half [of this three-season period has passed], the duration of the night equals that of the day. Eight [days after the spring, or vernal, equinox], the sound [of thunder] begins, and 10 [days after the autumnal equinox], it ceases.

"During the final third of winter and thereafter as the sun moves to the north, [the wind and sun] become exceedingly sharp, hot and rough, and by the power of these two elements, the qualities of the moon and earth [e.g. coolness and oiliness] are extinguished. At this time, the strong flavours of hotness, astringency and bitterness steal away the strength and vigour of human beings day by day.

"During the monsoon [and thereafter as the sun] proceeds southwards, one's strength again increases and the cool [quality of the earth] and the power of the moon are present, while [that of] the sun declines. Due to the falling of rain and the wind, the heat on the earth is pacified, and sour, salty and sweet flavours increase one's strength.

"Thus, the two periods of the movements [of the sun] have been revealed: in the winter [one's strength] is great, in the early and late summer, small, and in the autumn and spring, middling.

"Now [the discussion on] behaviour during the months and six seasons [is as follows]: due to the cold of early winter, the pores are blocked. As the digestive heat and [fire-accompanying] wind are strong, too little food will cause the physical constituents to decline. Thus one should eat [foods having] the first three flavours [of sourness, saltiness and sweetness]. During this time, one becomes hungry [in the early morning] due to the long nights, and this causes the physical constituents to decline [as the powerful digestive heat has nothing in the stomach upon which to act]. Thus sesamum oil [or other grain oils] should be rubbed [on the body], and one should [drink] meat broth and eat oily foods. Shoes and clothing to cover the skin should always be worn, and one should moderately warm oneself by a source of heat and the light of a fire and the sun. Dwell in houses made of earth and having double walls.

"As it is especially cold during the latter half of winter, following this behaviour is recommended. Phlegm is accumulated in the trunk of the body during the winter [because the winds in the body do not have passage through the pores, and the sun is weak, making the body cold]. In the spring, the light and warmth of the sun cause the digestive heat to decline. Phlegm disorders arise [as the digestive heat cannot digest as well], so one should eat [foods having] the latter three flavours [of bitterness, hotness and astringency]. Aged barley, the flesh of animals living in a dry environment, honey, boiled water and ginger soup—[in short] rough [food and drink]—should be consumed. Vigourous walking and rubbing lentil flour [on the skin] dispel phlegm disorders. Sit in the shadows of the sun in fragrant gardens and groves.

"As one's strength is lost due to the great heat of the rays of the sun during early summer, one should eat sweet, light, oily and cool [food]. Avoid salty, hot and sour [food] as well as physical exercise and staying put under the sun. Wash the body with cool water, and drink alcohol mixed with water [if one feels a need to take alcohol]. Wear very light clothing and dwell in a cool, fragrant house. Sit under shady trees and in places where a fragrant, moist breeze is blowing.

"Late summer, or monsoon, is moist due to water gathered in the clouds in the sky. The wind and cold, the steam from the earth, and muddy water harm the digestive heat, so one should apply means to increase it. Eat food having the first three flavours [of sourness, saltiness and sweetness] as well as food that is light, warm and oily. Drink alcohol made from grains planted in a dry region, and avoid staying in cool places [such as] on the roof of one's house.

"[The power of the rain and wind in] late summer is cool, but one's body is immediately scorched by the rays of the sun [when the clouds clear away]. The bile that accumulates during the monsoon [as a result of these conditions] arises in the autumn. In order to dispel this, one should eat [foods that are] sweet, bitter and astringent. Wear clothing that has been scented with camphor, sandalwood and ushi wood, and give the house a [cool, pleasant] aroma.

"In short, take warm food and drink during monsoon and winter, rough [nourishment] in the spring and cool [food] in early summer and autumn. During the monsoon and winter, take [foods having] the first three flavours [of sourness, saltiness and sweetness]; in the spring, use the latter three flavours [of bitterness, hotness and astringency]; and in the autumn, take sweet, bitter and astringent [foods]. During the autumn, take medicine to induce evacuation of the bowels [if there is an excess of bile], and during the spring, take medicine to induce vomiting [if there is an excess of phlegm]. In late summer, the use of enemas is recommended [for relieving wind disorders]. If [the conditions of the various seasons are] slight [e.g. little rain during the monsoon], excessive [e.g. extreme heat during early summer] or perverse [e.g. heat during the winter], give the appropriate treatment."

CHAPTER FIFTEEN

Occasional Behaviour

Then Sage Rigpé Yeshé spoke thus: "O great sage, listen! Thirdly, [the explanation of] occasional behaviour is [as follows]:

(III) "Do not obstruct the impulses of hunger, thirst, vomiting, yawning, sneezing, breathing, sleeping, [clearing the] mucus [from the throat], [removing excess] saliva [from the mouth and throat], excreting, [emitting] intestinal gas, urinating or [emitting] semen.

"Not satisfying hunger [causes] deterioration of the body, weakness, discomfort in the oesophagus after swallowing, and dizziness. As a remedy take [frequent] small quantities of light, oily and warm foods.

"Neglecting to satisfy one's thirst results in dryness of the mouth, dizziness, heart ailments and loss of mental clarity. For this all cool conditions [of nourishments, environment, etc.] are helpful.

"Suppressing [the need to] vomit leads to loss of appetite, discomfort in breathing, a disorder involving swelling of the eyes and skin combined with general paling (skya rbab), the appearance of many small itchy spots on the skin due to an increase of blood (me dbal), general itching (g-yan pa), chronic sores ('bras), leprosy, eye disorders, lung ailments and contagious diseases. Fasting, inhaling the smoke [of aloewood and sandalwood] and rinsing the mouth [with extracts from these woods are all methods that are of benefit in this case].

"By suppressing sneezing, the senses become unclear and one experiences headaches, stiffness of the neck in one direction, distortion of the mouth and loss of strength in the cheeks. [These effects are] dispelled by inhaling the smoke [of aloewood and sandalwood], using nasal medicine and looking at the sun.

> Nasal medicines are used in this manner. The patient lies down with his head lower than the rest of his body. Then four or five spoonfuls of the medicine are poured down his nostrils after blocking off the food passage in his throat with one's fingers. After five or 10 minutes, the

patient arises and the medicine in his nose together with many of the impurities in the nasal passages run out.

"Suppressing yawning gives similar effects [as those from suppressing sneezing], and these may be remedied by taking treatment to dispel wind disorders.

"Restraining the breath when one is exhausted leads to tumours, heart ailments and mental unclarity. [At such times], it is beneficial to rest and [take treatment to dispel] excess wind.

"Obstructing sleep causes much yawning, physical lassitude, heaviness of the head, visual unclarity and indigestion. Drinking meat broth and alcohol, rubbing the body (with oil) and sleeping are beneficial for such cases].

"Restraining [oneself from clearing] the mucus [from the throat] leads to an increase of throat mucus, discomfort in breathing, loss of weight, hiccoughs, heart ailments and discomfort in the oesophagus after swallowing. For this apply the means to remove throat mucus.

The best treatment for this is to drink a thick mixture of brown sugar, piper longum and ginger, all boiled together.

"Retaining [excess] saliva [in the throat and mouth] causes pain in the heart and head, falling of nasal fluid, dizziness and discomfort in the oesophagus after swallowing. Drinking alcohol, sleeping and holding pleasant conversations are beneficial for this.

"Obstructing the emission of intestinal gas causes dryness of the stool, blockage of intestinal gas and excrement, tumours and shooting pains [in the abdomen], weak eyesight, poor digestive heat and heart ailments.

"Obstructing defecation causes the rising of excrement into the mouth, pain in the brain, cramps, common colds and the ailments described above [as a result of obstructing intestinal gas].

"Obstructing urination brings about the formation of stones [in the kidneys and urinary bladder], ailments of the urinary organs, the male sex organ and the inside of the thighs as well as the above ailments [in the two previous cases]. The medication for this is of the type that is inserted into the sex organ, and one should also soak the body [in hot medicinal solutions], rub the body [with oil], apply hot or cold towels to the body and take vitamins.

"Blocking the emission of semen causes it to fall unintentionally and also leads to pain in the male sex organ, blockage of urine, increase of stones, and sexual impotence. One should [then] use medicines that are inserted into the sexual organ, soak the body [in hot medicinal solutions] and have intercourse with a woman. Also take sesamum oil, milk, chicken flesh and meat and drink alcohol.

"By obstructing these impulses and by forcefully acting upon them [e.g. sneezing with much force] all ailments arise and the winds are immediately disturbed. Therefore, use [the appropriate] food, medicine and liquid as remedies. Although a disorder may be relieved by fasting and pacifying [it with the proper medication], it will arise [again like] a corpse, but not if [the body is] well purified. Therefore, [take medicine to induce vomiting] to purify the cold disorders in the spring, [which come as a result of the phlegm accumulated in the winter. During the monsoon, [use enemas to] purify [the body of wind disorders that come from the] accumulation [of wind during] early summer. In the autumn, [take medicine to evacuate the bowels, thereby] purifying [the body of excess bile that has] accumulated during the monsoon.

"Good purification makes for a complete cure and an absence of ailments. If one continually takes wholesome food, follows healthy behaviour and goes to an experienced physician, one will not become ill. For the prevention of the arising of all disorders and the pacification of those that have arisen, following these patterns of behaviour [on the suitable] occasions is recommended."

****

Appendix

The following are examples of foods bearing the various inherent and secondary qualities.

Inherent Qualities

1 heaviness: potato, corn, wheat
2 oiliness: eggs, the flesh of water-dwelling animals, mango, banana, pomegranate
3 coolness: cauliflower, cabbage, pork
4 softening agent: spinach
5 lightness: poultry, the flesh of four-legged animals
6 roughness: coffee, rabbit flesh, the flesh of carnivorous animals
7 heat: buffalo meat, pomegranate
8 acridity: hot chilli.

Secondary Qualities

1 gentleness: foods grown in a moist, windy environment
2 heaviness: bone marrow, potatoes, cabbage
3 warmth: hot chilli, pomegranate
4 oiliness: sesamum oil and other grain oils, yak meat
5 firmness: rabbit brain and other foods that counteract diarrhoea
6 coldness: foods grown in a windy environment
7 softening agent: spinach and other foods grown in an environment having a strong element of earth
8 coolness: orange, vegetables in general
9 pliability: foods grown in water
10 thinness [of fluids]: foods grown in water
11 dryness: foods grown in a hot, dry environment
12 fatlessness: pulses and other foods with little or no fat content
13 heat: foods grown in a hot, sunny environment
14 lightness: foods grown in a cool, windy environment
15 acridity: foods grown in a sunny, dry environment
16 roughness: foods grown in a dry, windy environment
17 motility: foods grown in a windy environment.

Glossary

aloewood: *a ga ru*
asthma: *dbugs mi bde ba*
bile, accomplishing: *mkhris pa sgrub byed*
    colour-transforming: *mkhris pa mdangs sgyur*
    complexion-clearing: *mkhris pa mdog gsal*
    digestive: *mkhris pa 'ju byed*
    visually-operating: *mkhris pa mthong byed*
bones, pelvic: *mtshang ra*
Capsicum annum: *tsi tra ka*
channel: *rtsa*
channel of connections: *'brel ba'i rtsa*
    of existence: *srid pa'i rtsa*
    of formation: *chags pa'i rtsa*
    of life: *tshe yi rtsa*
channel, central: *rtsa 'u ma*
    vital: *srog rtsa*
chyle: *dvangs ma*
constituents, bodily: *lus zungs*
cord, spinal: *klad gzhung*
Crataegus pinnatifid ı: *skyur ru*
Crataegus sanguinea: *ba ru ra*
disease, venereal: *reg pa'i dug*
Elettaria cardamomum: *sug smel*
Gentiana barbata: *tig ta*
goitre: *lba ba*
gout: *dreg nad*
haemorrhoids: *gzhang 'brum*
Hemerocallis minor : *gser gyi me tog*
hipbone: *dpyi*
Hippophae rhamnoides: *star bu*
humour: *nad, nyes pa*
impurities: *dri ma*
intestine, large: *long*
    small: *sgyu ma*
jaw bone: *mur 'gram*

ligament, large: *chu ba*
      small: *rgyus pa*
lymph: *chur ser*
Mesua roxburgii: *na le sham*
nutriment, essential: *bcud*
   regenerative: *khu ba*
   vesicle of regenerative: *bsam seu*
oil, body: *zhag*
organs, five solid: *don lnga*
   six hollow: *snod drug*
phlegm, connecting: *bad kan 'byor byed*
   experiencing: *bad kan myong byed*
   mixing: *bad kan tshim byed*
   satisfying: *bad kan tshim byed*
   supportive: *bad kan rten byed*
Piper longum: *pi pi ling*
plasma: *phyi sa*
pox: *'brum bu*
Pterospermum acerifolium: *dong ga*
quality, inherent: *nus pa*
   secondary: *yon dan*
Rhododendron anthropogonoides maxim.: *da lis*
Santalum album: *tsan dan*
scrotum: *gsang sgro*
sediment, inferior: *snyigs ma*
spine, base of : *rked pa*
Tantra: Explanatory: *bSHad rgyud*
   Oral Tradition: *Man ngag gi rgyud*
   Root: *rTSa rgyud*
   Subsequent: *PHyi ma'i rgyud*
Terminalia chebula: *a ru*
tumour: *skran*
vertebra: *sgal tshigs 'phang lo*
vessel, blood: *rtsa nag*
   lymphatic: *rtsa dkar*
wind, downward-clearing: *rlung thur sel*
   fire-accompanying: *rlung me mnyam*
   life-supporting: *rlung srog 'dzin*
   pervasive: *rlung khyab byed*
   upward-moving: *rlung gyen rgyu*